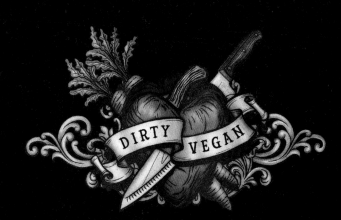

DIRTY VEGAN

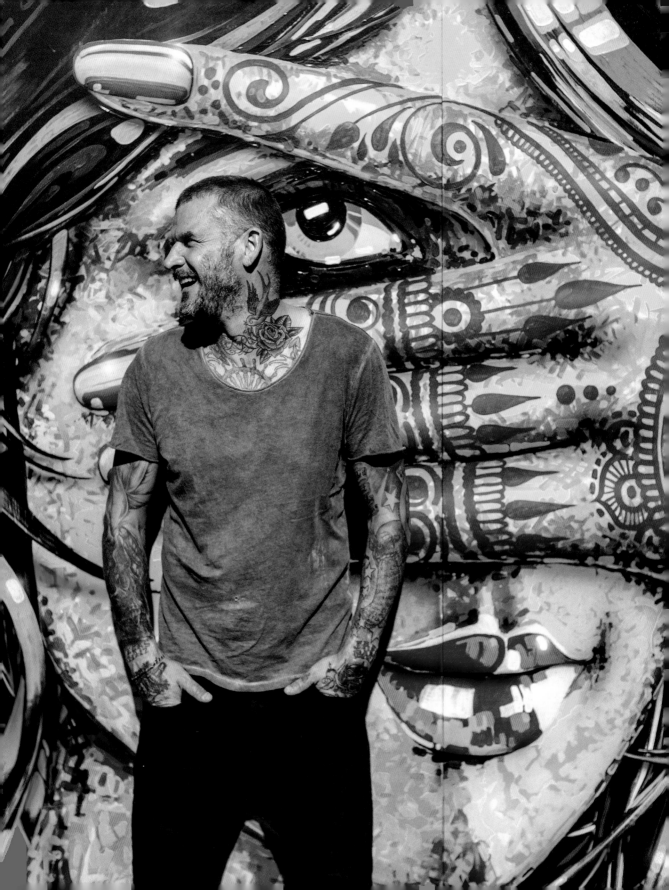

DIRTY VEGAN ANOTHER BITE

Matt Pritchard

BRAND-NEW ROCKING VEGAN RECIPES

MITCHELL BEAZLEY

FOR THE ANIMALS

An Hachette UK Company
www.hachette.co.uk

First published in Great Britain in 2019 by Mitchell Beazley,
an imprint of Octopus Publishing Group Ltd
Carmelite House, 50 Victoria Embankment, London EC4Y 0DZ
www.octopusbooks.co.uk

Text copyright © One Tribe TV Limited 2019
Design and layout copyright © Octopus Publishing Group 2019

ISBN 978-1-78472-630-0

A CIP catalogue record for this book is available from the British Library.

Printed and bound in Italy

10 9 8 7 6 5 4 3 2 1

Editorial Director Eleanor Maxfield
Senior Editor Sophie Elletson
Design and Art Direction Smith & Gilmour
Photographer (portraits) Chris Terry
Photographer (food) Jamie Orlando Smith
Food Stylist Phil Mundy
Props Stylist Olivia Wardle
Cover Illustrator Andy Smith
Creative Director Jonathan Christie
Production Manager Caroline Alberti
Recipe development lead Bob Andrew
Additional recipe development Anna Shepherd
Head of Brand for Dirty Vegan/One Tribe TV Rachel Lovell

CONTENTS

PREFACE 9

EASY MIDWEEK FILLERS 12

BALANCED and BANGING 40

HOME COMFORT CLASSICS 68

FOOD WITH LEGS 96

SWEET STUFF 124

DINNER WITH MATES 158

ACKNOWLEDGEMENTS 202

INDEX 204

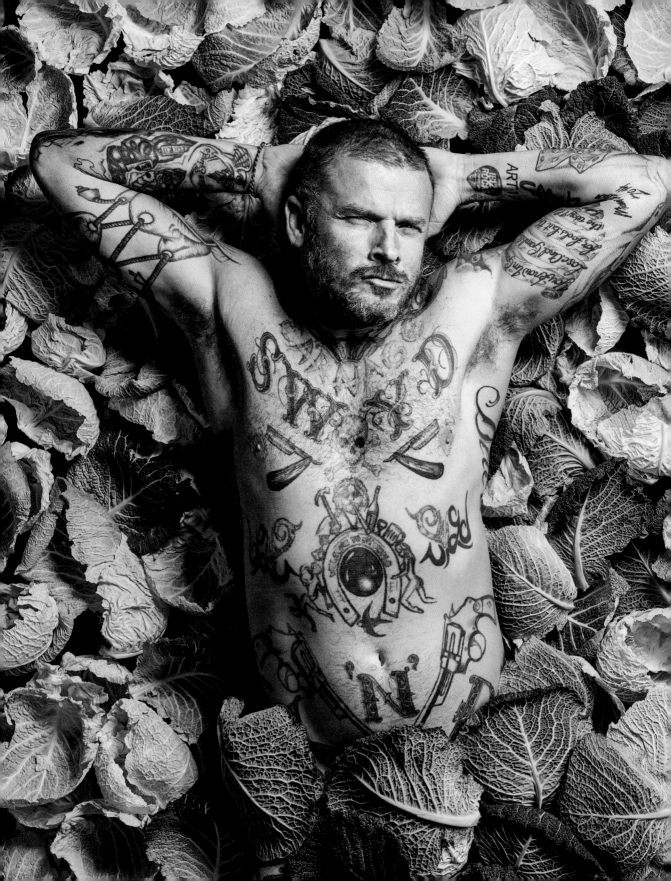

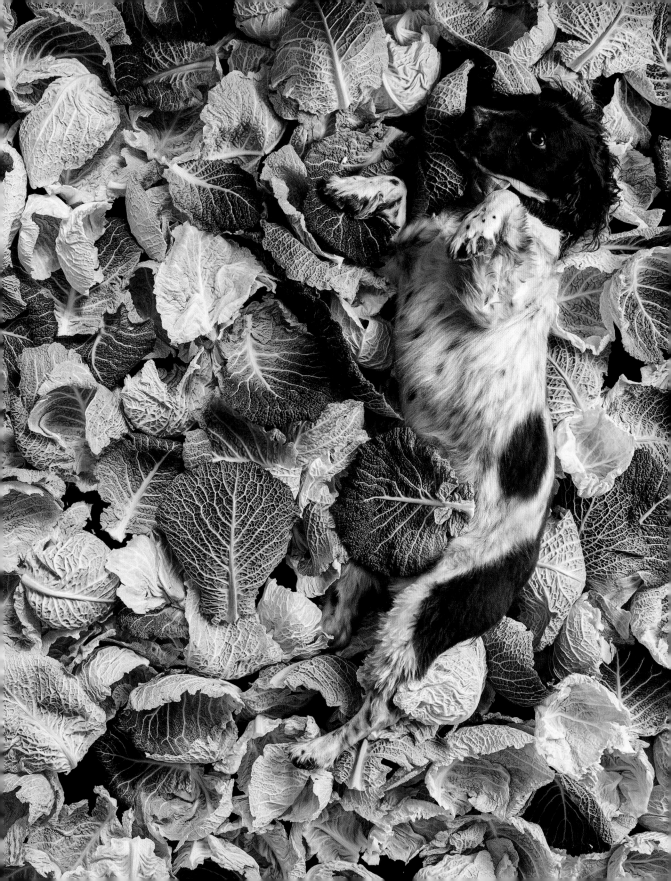

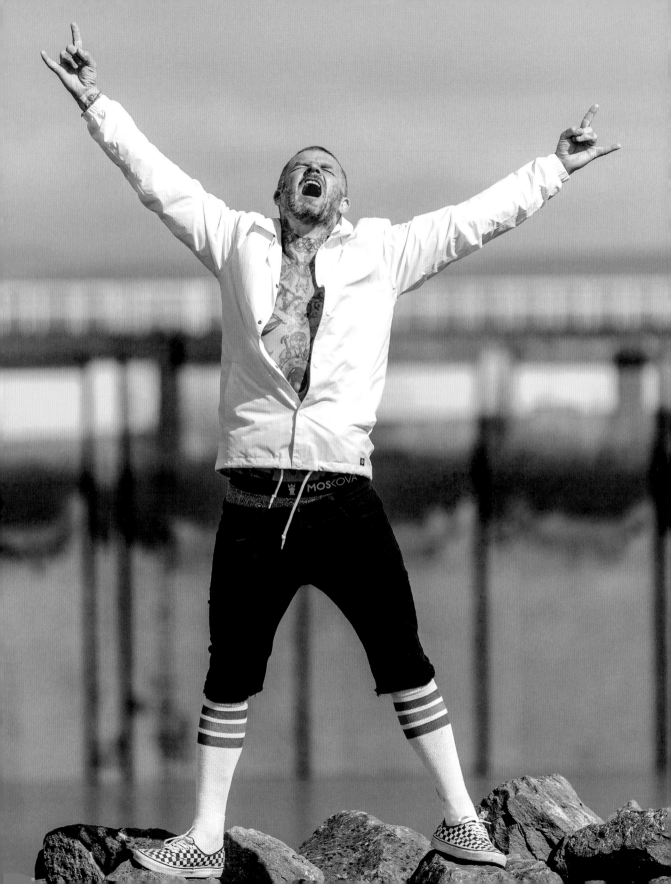

★ PREFACE ★

Welcome to my second cookery book! Just writing that sentence spins me out – I never dreamed I would have one cookbook, let alone two. Whether you are just trying to cut down on meat and dairy, or want to go fully vegan, this book is for you. The recipes are designed to make plant-based cooking and eating (and I do mean both) as enjoyable as possible. No mysterious ingredients or methods, no fancy-pants cheffiness and – on the whole – avoiding processed ingredients.

Don't get me wrong, I reckon a sprinkling of vegan cheese or a helping of meat alternative is all good (as you'll see from my comfort foods chapter), I just don't think we should eat them all the time. So the starting point with all these recipes is veg, veg, veg… and loads of it! I reckon the more natural your diet, the better off you'll be. If you're like me and you enjoy a bit of junk (crisps are my weak point), just follow the 80 : 20 rule (be good 80 per cent of the time).

As with my first book, *Dirty Vegan*, I've worked with Bob Andrew, an amazing chef in Devon who is a total veg expert, to make sure these recipes are surprising and different, easy to make, overflowing with the green stuff and – most of all – proper tasty. Start with the Roasting Tin Laksa, Sticky Tofu Bao Buns and the Rhubarb and Custard Doughnuts if you want to get straight into my favourites (*see* pages 25, 108 and 136)! Make sure you give the Dinner with Mates chapter a go, too (*see* pages 158–201). Nothing brings people together like food does, and it seems that spending time with the people we care about has become harder than ever these days with our busy lives, so don't wait for an excuse, just invite everyone round and get in the kitchen.

For those who don't know my story, I grew up in Cardiff with my brothers and my mam and dad and had a pretty normal childhood, though my eccentricity did surface now and then! It was in my early twenties that my life really changed. I'd been obsessed with skateboarding since school and turned pro when I got spotted by a scout who'd seen me win a competition. Me and my mate Dainton started mixing skateboarding with pranks and dares, filming them as we went. We released a video of our messing about and it went mental… to cut a long story short, MTV called us up and that is where *Dirty Sanchez* began. Ten years of craziness ensued, and while I had the best time (a lot of which I can't remember), the partying and rock 'n' roll lifestyle eventually caught up with me in the form of awful, awful depression. It was switching my addiction from booze and drugs to fitness that got me out of it, and by constantly challenging myself to physical tests of endurance, I have found I can keep clear of the darkness most of the time.

It was through becoming an ultra-athlete that I flipped the vegan switch. I kept reading that lots of triathletes and ironman champions were vegan, so at first that was my motivation. When I looked into veganism more, the environmental argument against meat and dairy seemed so strong as to be irresistible. I became fully vegan four years ago and have not looked back. I started the *Pritchards' Proper Vegan Cookin'* YouTube channel and then the BBC came knocking.

Since the launch of my first book and the BBC cookery series *Dirty Vegan*, it's been a mental year and I've learned a lot. Even though I studied at catering college in my younger days, I've been out of the game for a long time and it's only thanks to the help of many people, especially Bob Andrew and Laura from Tidy Kitchen in Cardiff, that I've been able to build on my plant-based cooking. I've got in the kitchen for a lot of events, and cooking for big numbers of diners was a right eyeopener, but I absolutely loved it. Laura and I made a few recipes from my book in a restaurant in Manchester and that was my first time back in a pro kitchen for many years. We were pressed to get the dishes out in time... and it was that pressure that I loved! We managed to send every course out and I got to mingle with the diners for a chat and to see what they thought of the food. Everyone left with happy faces, which is a great feeling.

I also cooked at the Riverford restaurant in Devon for 70 people. I spent all day working alongside Bob, prepping for the evening's meal. That day was a reminder of what hard work really is, but I wasn't moaning: to cook alongside someone who has such an amazing knowledge of all things green was so rewarding. When customers started arriving for drinks, my nerves kicked in, as I had to give a talk before the meal. It might sound daft to those who know me from my *Dirty Sanchez* days, but I'm actually quite shy! In the end, the food was perfect, so was the service and my nerves relaxed just in time for my Q & A session with the diners. It was a great day and everyone made me feel so welcome. To say we earned

a good few beers in the local after was an understatement, but they always taste so much better when you've earned them.

I also had my first cooking demo. Yep, cooking in front of a load of people up in Scotland with a sharp knife in my hand and a gas stove at my back... complete with nerves, of course. I was thinking: how can I pull this off? I'm fine cooking in a normal kitchen, as I find it therapeutic, but to cook in front of others is a whole new ball game. Bob had done quite a few demos in the past, so gave me some great advice. I practised in my house a few times, but, at the end of the day, you just turn up, make the demo your own and add your own little pzazz. I felt more confident cooking in front of a crowd than I did just doing a talk. I have a load more demos lined up and I really feel I can give the audience a good laugh now!

Since my first book was published and the BBC series hit the screens, I've finally invested in my dream kitchen. I've wanted one for many years and now seemed the perfect time to get it, as I'll be spending a great deal of time in it prepping and cooking great new dishes to share with you all. The rollercoaster life I once led, which was heaps of fun, has now returned me to where I started many years ago at catering college: I'm back in the kitchen. I love it and I can't wait to bring you more vegan dishes.

I hope you have fun with this book. Use it to feed your family. Get your mates round. Or just cook to relax and feed yourself. Everyone deserves decent food. Here's to healthy plant-based grub and all the good it brings!

MATT PRITCHARD
Skateboarder, Ultra-athlete, Cook

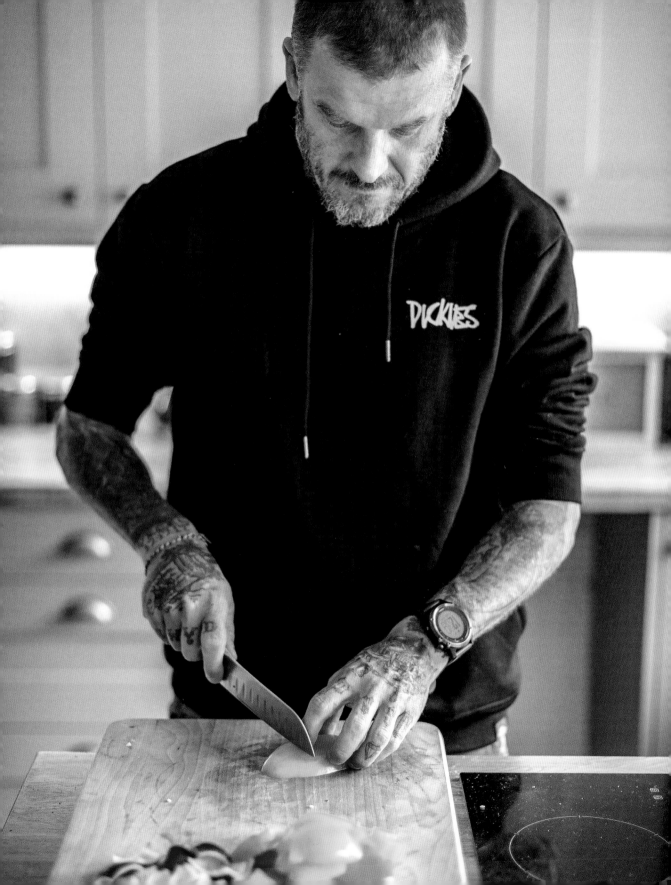

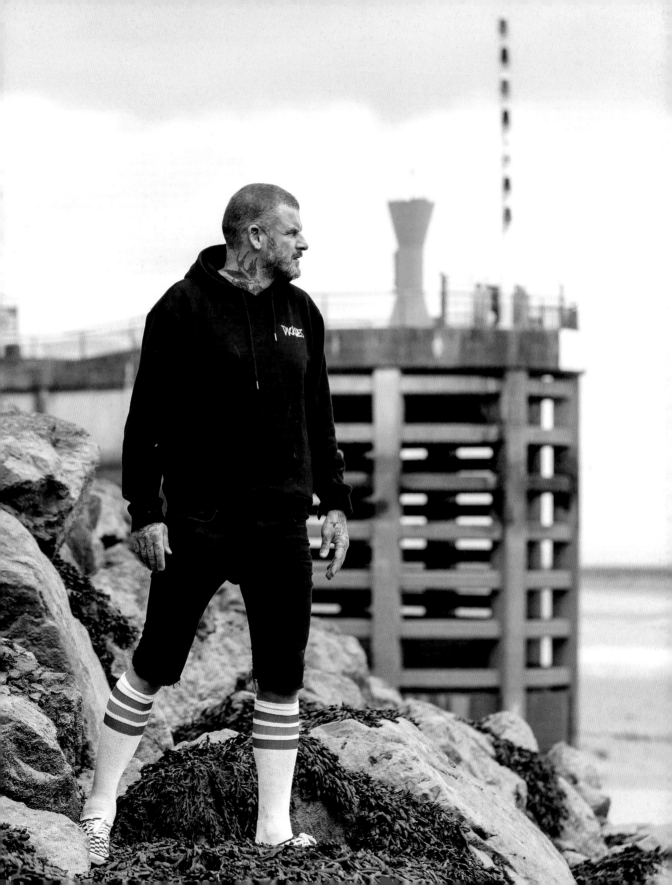

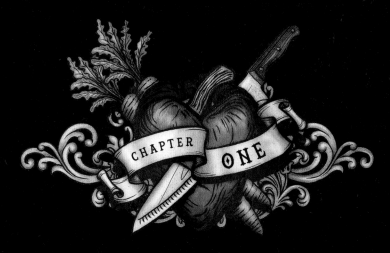

CHAPTER ONE

EASY MIDWEEK FILLERS

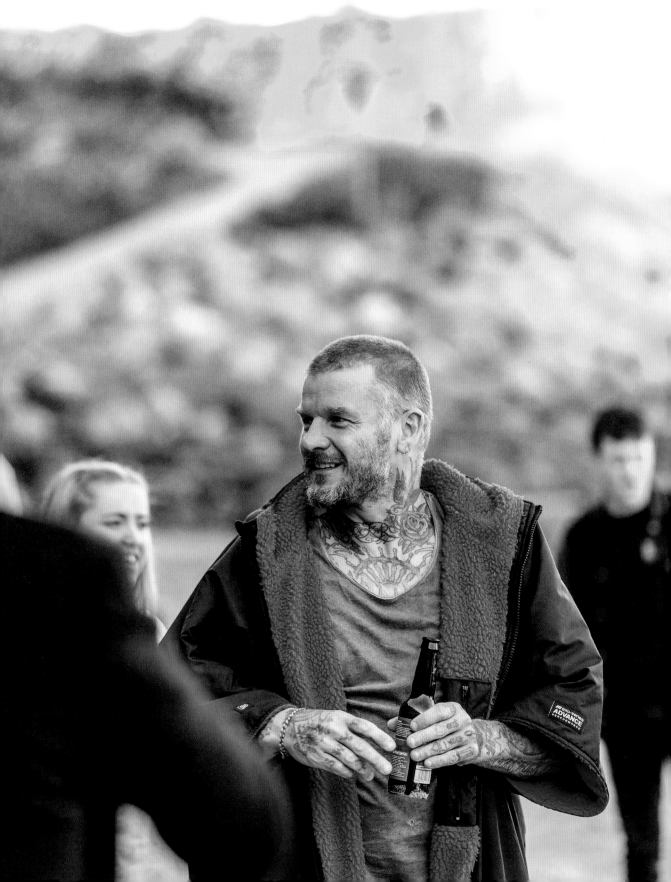

Comparing my behaviour during the height of my chaotic *Dirty Sanchez* touring days with how I look after myself now is mind-blowing. From the moment we left home it was carnage until we got back a few weeks or months later. My eating routine went entirely out of the window… in fact – if I'm honest – eating happened very rarely, due to the daily use of narcotics, alcohol and cigarettes and a general lack of sleep.

I'll never forget jumping on a proper tour bus for the first time, as excited as a kid in a sweet shop, looking forward to spending time with my three good friends, travelling all over the country doing gigs of our live show. This big dude Johnny B, our tour manager, introduced himself with a firm handshake and proceeded to explain the tour rules and the dos and don'ts of the bus. I always remember he said, 'In the mornings I'll make a big saucepan of porridge for everyone,' and, at that point, I thought he might have been our butler, too! There were stoves on the bus, but they were only really used when Johnny made porridge. The microwave worked hard, though, heating up pasties for us. The boys all knew I had a culinary background, so sometimes would joke about me cooking everyone a meal, but to be honest I was never in a state to be able to. A knife in my hand back then would have been dangerous.

On the road, my priorities were:

1. Alcohol
2. Narcotics
3. Cigarettes
4. Music
5. Food

Yep, food was last on the list and every time we *did* eat it was service station rubbish: overpriced crisps, sandwiches and bottom-of-the-barrel pasties. Johnny B's porridge was always served when I was at the back of the bus, rocking out to Kiss's 'Rock and roll all nite' in a right pickle, and I see now that he was making sure we got some basic fuel in our bodies at the right moment; it probably made all the difference, as I didn't eat much else! You see, when we were on the road, the day started when we woke up at 5pm, we got on stage at 9pm, then we partied until we dropped… until it was time to do it all again.

How times change, eh? Little did I know then that I'd one day be writing my second vegan cookbook. It's so far from what I once used to be, but I wouldn't change what I've become for the world. When I'm busy these days, I always find a way to eat well and get something decent inside my body. The same should apply whether you work in an office or have a really physical job: don't forget that food is fuel, and the better the fuel the better your daily performance will be. But it should also be tasty! I know it's hard to get stuck into cooking when you come home from work knackered, but I hope this collection of simple recipes will help.

Welcome to my easy midweek meals. I hope you enjoy cooking them… and eating them!

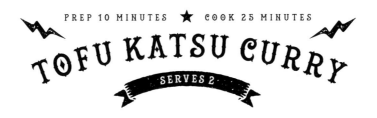

TOFU KATSU CURRY

SERVES 2

For the curry sauce
2 tablespoons vegetable oil
1 small onion, finely chopped
1 carrot, grated
1 garlic clove, finely chopped
1 tablespoon medium
    curry powder
1 tablespoon plain flour
400ml hot water
pinch of sugar (optional)
salt

For the tofu
3 tablespoons cornflour
3 tablespoons cold water
60g panko breadcrumbs
200g marinated tofu
flavourless vegetable oil

To serve
jasmine rice, cooked according
    to the packet instructions
handful of shredded vegetables
    (spring onions, carrots,
    cucumbers, radishes and sugar
    snap peas all jump to mind),
    or salad leaves dressed with
    a little lime juice

A katsu is a strange dish; it hardly feels Japanese at all. The sauce is fairly mild and inoffensive and reminds me of the curry sauce you get slathered over hot chips in a late-night takeaway... you can take that as an alternative serving suggestion! Marinated tofu is easy to buy in most supermarkets, but if you can't find it, just marinate some plain tofu in a bit of soy, tamari or teriyaki sauce overnight.

Start the curry sauce by heating the oil in a saucepan. Cook the onion, carrot and garlic with a pinch of salt over a medium-low heat for 10 minutes, until starting to soften. Add the curry powder and flour and cook for a further 2 minutes, then gradually add the water in small amounts, stirring as you go to avoid lumps. Simmer for 10 minutes, then blend until smooth. You may want to thin it with a bit more water, it should have the consistency of a thick soup. Taste and adjust the seasoning with more salt and a pinch of sugar, if you think it needs it. Set aside.

For the tofu, mix the cornflour and cold water in a shallow bowl to make a sticky paste. Tip the breadcrumbs into a second bowl. Slice the tofu in half horizontally, so you have 2 flat squares. Turn them in the cornflour mix to coat, then turn them in the breadcrumbs until completely covered.

Heat a 5mm depth of oil in a high-sided frying pan. Fry the tofu for 2–3 minutes a side, until golden.

Reheat the sauce and spoon it next to the freshly cooked jasmine rice on warm plates. Cut the tofu into thick slices and perch it on top, so it doesn't get soggy, and serve with the shredded raw veg or lime-dressed salad leaves.

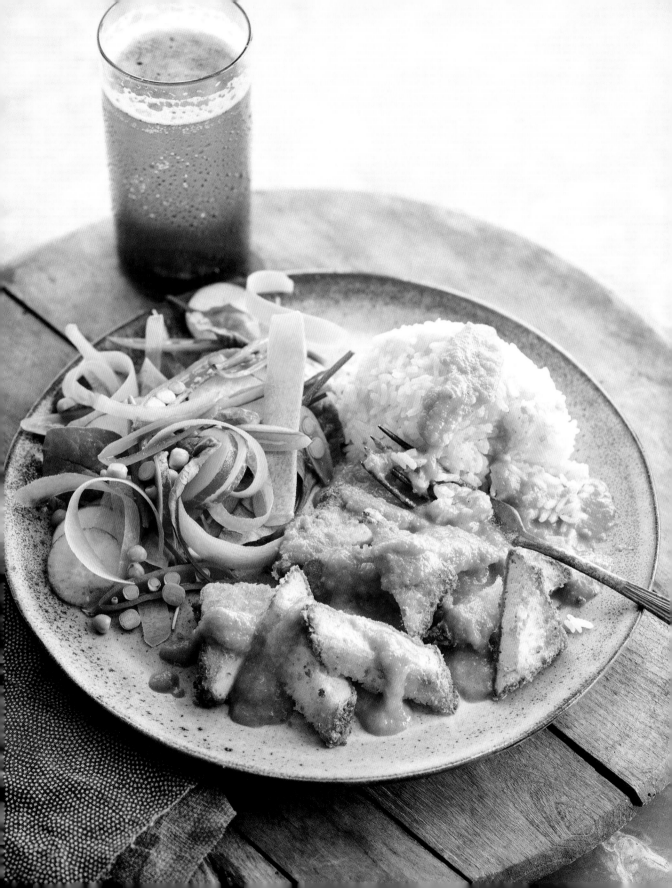

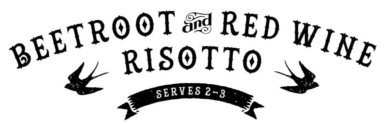

BEETROOT and RED WINE RISOTTO

SERVES 2~3

2 tablespoons olive oil
1 red onion, finely chopped
1 celery stick, finely chopped
2 large beetroots, peeled
   and grated
1 garlic clove, finely chopped
1 teaspoon chopped
   rosemary leaves
200g arborio rice
175ml red wine
800ml hot vegetable stock
   (see page 121 for homemade)
2 tablespoons nutritional yeast
30g walnuts, toasted and chopped
leaves from a small bunch of
   parsley, chopped
salt and pepper

VARIATIONS

Forget the walnuts and parsley and try finishing the dish with freshly grated horseradish and chopped dill instead, for a Scandi feel.

Toasted and chopped hazelnuts could replace the walnuts, along with some finely grated orange zest and a wee squeeze of the juice.

Add half a finely chopped fennel bulb with the onion and celery. The aniseed taste isn't for everyone, but I think it is cracking with beetroot. Any fronds can be chopped and sprinkled on top at the end.

Not a dish to eat when wearing a white T-shirt, or on a first date. Risottos are usually made with white wine; that would work equally well here taste-wise, but red wine seems more in keeping with the colour scheme, plus it adds a wintry, stew-like taste. You could use pearled spelt or barley instead of rice; they'll plump up in much the same way but may take a little more time and stock to cook.

Warm the olive oil in a large saucepan. Add the onion, celery, grated beetroot and a pinch of salt. Cook gently for 10 minutes, until starting to soften.

Add the garlic, rosemary and rice. Cook for 2 more minutes, before tipping in the red wine. Let it cook away until the wine has been absorbed by the rice.

Reduce the heat to medium-low and add a ladle of hot stock. Cook gently, stirring often, until the stock has been absorbed. Add another ladle of stock and repeat until the rice is tender; this will take 20–25 minutes.

Let the risotto rest for 5 minutes, then stir in the nutritional yeast until dissolved. Taste and tweak the seasoning with salt and pepper, then serve sprinkled with the walnuts and parsley.

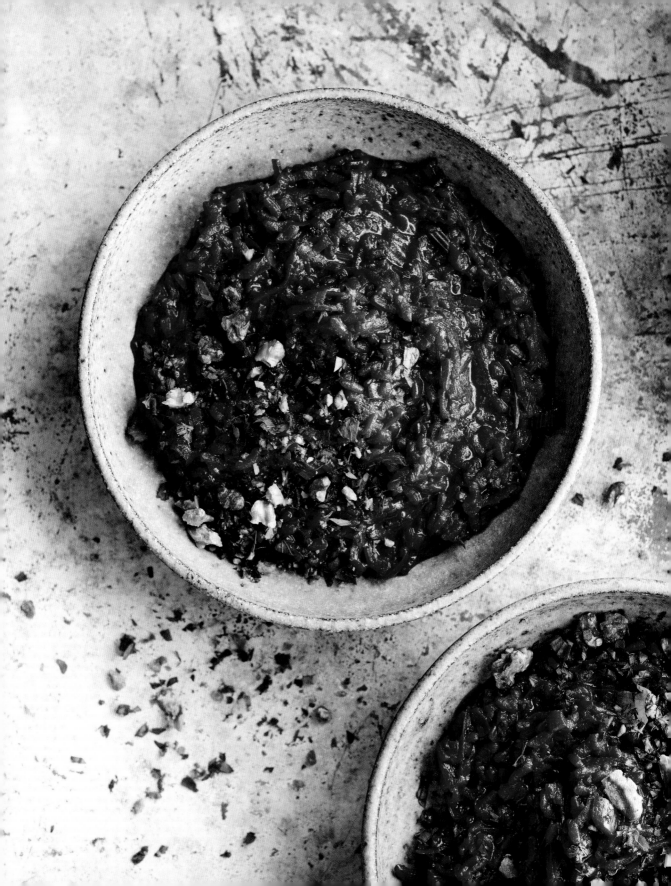

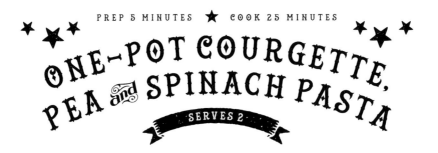

ONE-POT COURGETTE, PEA and SPINACH PASTA

SERVES 2

2 tablespoons olive oil,
   plus extra to serve
2 courgettes, grated
   or very thinly sliced
1 unwaxed lemon
2 garlic cloves, finely chopped
125ml white wine
300ml light vegetable stock
   (*see* page 121 for homemade)
200ml unsweetened almond milk
200g penne pasta
100g frozen peas
100g baby spinach
leaves from a small bunch
   of parsley, chopped
a few mint leaves, chopped
2 tablespoons nutritional yeast
   (optional)
salt and pepper

A bowl of the green stuff! The trick to finishing a good pasta sauce is to add a dash of the pasta cooking water at the end, as the starch it contains adds a slight creaminess. This dish takes that logic to its extreme conclusion by cooking the pasta in the sauce, using just enough liquid to cook it. As the water is absorbed, the starch turns the courgettes into a rich, glossy sauce. As long as the liquid-to-pasta ratios are correct, you can adapt this technique endlessly, using whatever veg you have to hand.

Warm the olive oil in a large saucepan. Add the courgettes and a good pinch of salt. Cook gently over a medium-low heat for 10 minutes, until the courgettes start to soften.

Finely zest half the lemon and add it to the pan along with the garlic and white wine. Let the mixture bubble away until the wine has evaporated.

Tip in the stock and milk, bring to the boil, then add the pasta and peas. Reduce the heat to a simmer, pop on a lid and simmer for 12 minutes, or until the pasta is nearly cooked.

Remove the lid, stir in the spinach and cook for a further 2 minutes. Fold the parsley and mint into the pan, then taste and tweak with salt, pepper and a generous squeeze or so of lemon juice.

Pile into warm shallow bowls and finish with a drizzle of good olive oil. You can sprinkle with a little nutritional yeast as a Parmesan substitute, if you like.

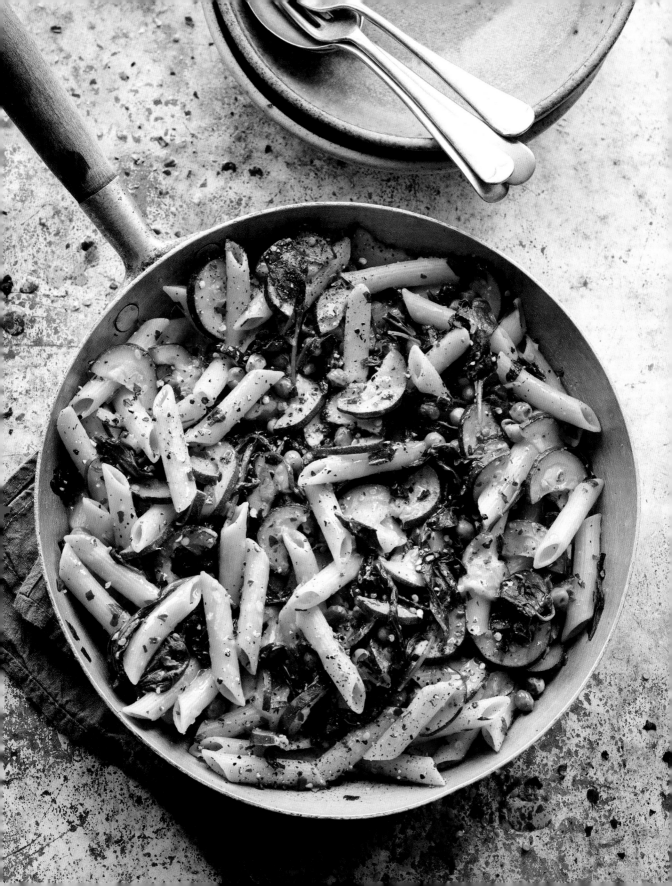

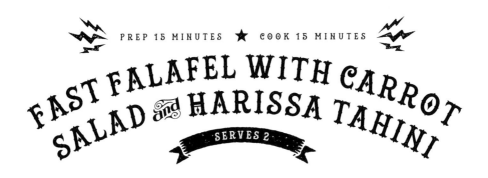

FAST FALAFEL WITH CARROT SALAD and HARISSA TAHINI

SERVES 2

For the falafel (to make 8)
400g can chickpeas, drained
1 garlic clove
1 teaspoon ground cumin
1 teaspoon ground coriander
small bunch of parsley
small bunch of coriander
1 tablespoon plain flour
3 tablespoons olive oil
salt and pepper

For the salad
2 carrots, sliced into ribbons
   with a vegetable peeler
½ red onion, thinly sliced
¼ teaspoon ground
   cardamom seeds
1 teaspoon poppy seeds
4–6 mint leaves, torn
1 tablespoon olive oil
1 lemon

For the harissa tahini
3 tablespoons tahini
1 tablespoon harissa
1 tablespoon olive oil
4 tablespoons boiling water

To serve
4 pitta breads
80g bag good-quality
   mixed salad leaves

A vegan standard, but given a banging lift! The ingredients list looks long, but it is faster than you'd think to put together. Tahini acts strangely when you try to make the sauce; it will look like it is thickening and splitting at the start, but have faith and stay with it, as it will come together in the end.

Preheat the oven to 160°C (Gas Mark 3).

Throw all the falafel ingredients except the oil into a food processor, season well with salt and pepper and blitz into a coarse paste. Shape the mix into 8 equal-sized balls (it's easier to do this if you wet your hands first). Slightly flatten each ball to form a burger shape. Heat the olive oil in a frying pan. Fry the falafels for 2–3 minutes a side, until golden. Transfer them to the oven for 10 minutes.

Meanwhile, mix the carrots, red onion, cardamom, poppy seeds and mint in a bowl. Add the olive oil, a good squeeze of lemon juice and a pinch of salt. Taste and tweak the seasoning: you may want more lemon juice, or more salt.

To make the sauce, mix the tahini with the harissa and olive oil. Gradually add the boiling water, whisking and adding more if needed, until it reaches a thick yogurt-like consistency. Season well with salt.

Toast or grill the pitta breads and split them along one side. Fill them with salad leaves, some carrot salad and a generous slick of tahini sauce. Wedge 2 hot falafels into each and scoff immediately, with as much grace as you can.

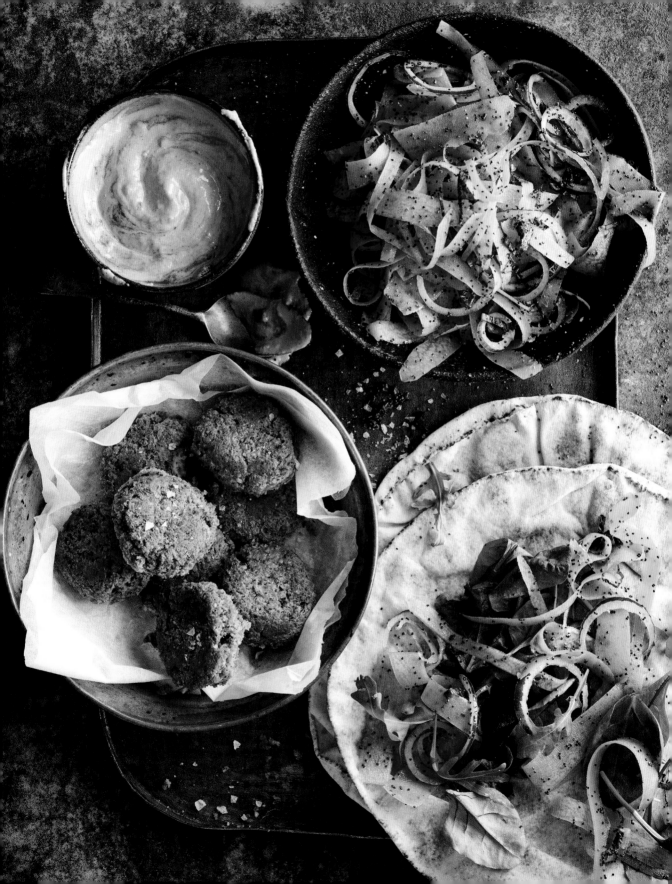

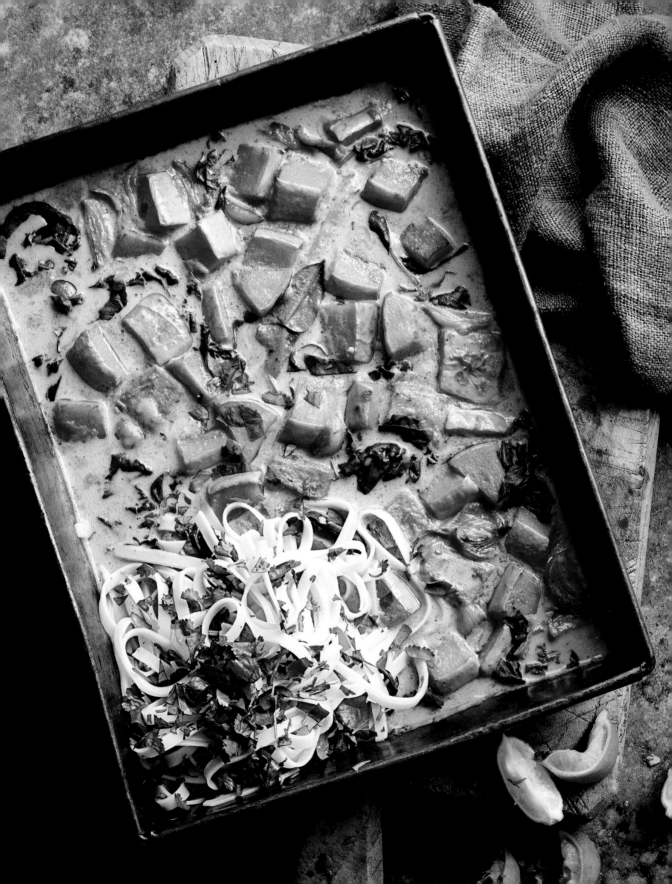

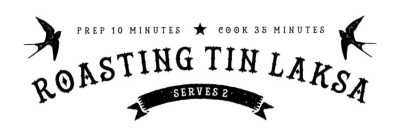

ROASTING TIN LAKSA

SERVES 2

500g squash, chopped
    into 2cm chunks
4 shallots, cut into wedges
vegetable oil
400g can coconut milk
300ml vegetable stock
    (*see page 121 for homemade*)
1 lemon grass stalk
4 lime leaves
100g rice noodles
100g baby spinach
small handful of coriander
    leaves, roughly chopped
salt and pepper
lime wedges, to serve

For the laksa paste
1 teaspoon ground cumin
1 teaspoon ground turmeric
1 tablespoon finely grated
    fresh root ginger
1 garlic clove
3 red bird's eye chillies,
    stalk ends cut off
1 tablespoon soy sauce
dash of flavourless vegetable oil
    (optional)

This is a hearty bowl of South East Asian-inspired noodles – bang on for a midweek feed. The broth is usually made in a pan but, since squash roasted in a tin always seems to taste better, I make it in the oven. If you can't be bothered to blend your own paste, you can use a few tablespoons of Thai red curry paste instead.

Preheat the oven to 200°C (Gas Mark 6). Place the squash and shallots in a roasting tin and oil and season them well. Pop into the oven to roast for 20 minutes.

Meanwhile, make the laksa paste by blending all the ingredients together in a small food processor. Alternatively, bash them together in a mortar and pestle, adding a dash of oil if it has difficulty coming together.

When the squash and shallots have had 20 minutes, stir in the laksa paste, coconut milk and stock. Give the lemon grass stalk a bash to split it open and throw that into the tray along with the lime leaves. Return to the oven for a further 10–15 minutes, until the squash is tender.

Meanwhile, cook the noodles in a saucepan of salted boiling water according to the packet instructions. Cool immediately in cold water and drain well.

Remove the roasting tin from the oven and pluck out the lemon grass and lime leaves. Stir in the spinach to wilt.

Divide the cold noodles between 2 warm deep bowls. Ladle the laksa broth over the top, sprinkle with the coriander and serve with lime wedges for squeezing.

MUSHROOM RAGÚ and POLENTA

SERVES 2

For the ragú

2 tablespoons olive oil
1 onion, finely chopped
1 celery stick, finely chopped
400g mixed mushrooms, sliced
    (see recipe introduction)
2 garlic cloves, finely chopped
1 bay leaf
2 thyme sprigs
200g tomatoes, chopped
175ml white wine
200ml vegetable stock,
    preferably dark and with
    mushrooms (see page 121)
leaves from a small bunch
    of parsley, chopped
salt and pepper

For the polenta

400ml unsweetened plant-based
    milk, plus extra if needed
100g quick-cook polenta
2 tablespoons nutritional yeast
2 tablespoons olive oil

This dish is best made when the season is right and you can get your hands on some wild, foraged 'shrooms, though it is just as easily made with a selection of chestnuts and Portobellos. Polenta can be deeply comforting, on a par with a bowl of mash or pasta, but it is a blank canvas and will only taste as bold as the seasoning you add.

Heat the olive oil in a frying pan and cook the onion and celery over a medium-low heat for 10 minutes, until starting to soften. Increase the heat and add the mushrooms with a good pinch of salt. Fry for 5 minutes until starting to colour, then add the garlic, bay, thyme, tomatoes and wine and let the mixture bubble away until reduced by half. Tip in the stock, reduce the heat to a simmer and cook for 10 minutes.

Meanwhile, make the polenta. Pour the milk into a saucepan with a pinch of salt and bring it to a simmer. (You may need more or less liquid, depending on the brand you are using, so check the packet instructions.) Pour in the polenta in a steady stream, stirring as you do. Return to a simmer, stirring well for about 2 minutes, or until the mixture thickens and comes away from the sides of the pan. Remove from the heat and stir in the nutritional yeast and olive oil. You might want to loosen with a dash more milk; the consistency should be somewhere between soft mash and thick porridge. Taste and season with salt and pepper.

Taste the ragú and tweak the seasoning. Fish out the bay and thyme stalks, if you can. Spoon generous dollops of polenta into warm shallow bowls, top with the ragú and sprinkle with parsley.

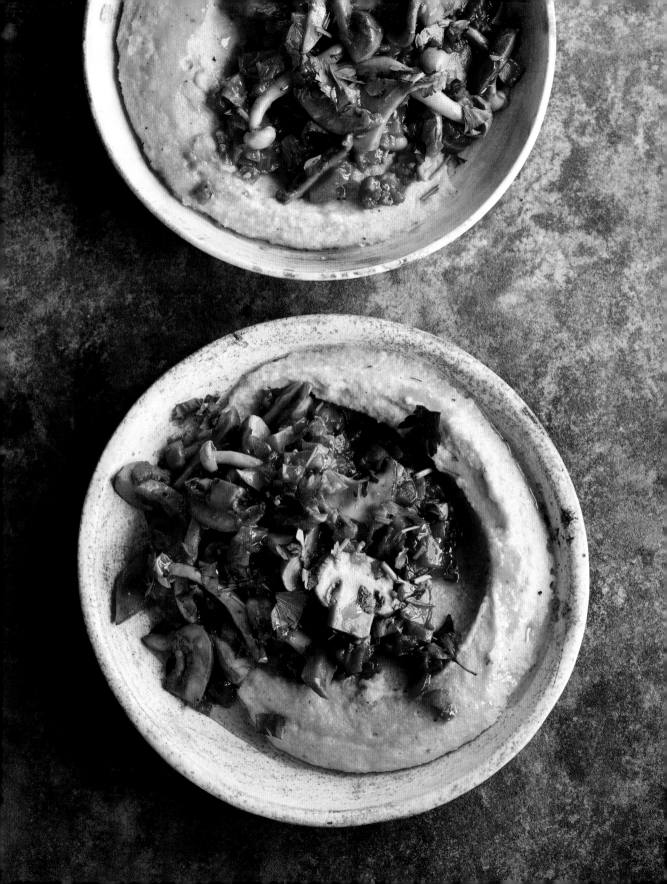

PEKING CRISPY JACKFRUIT PANCAKES

SERVES 2

For the pancakes
400g can baby jackfruit
3 tablespoons soy sauce
½ teaspoon Chinese five spice
1 tablespoon rice vinegar
½ teaspoon crushed
   Szechuan pepper
2 tablespoons untoasted
   sesame oil
½ cucumber
3 spring onions
10–12 Chinese pancakes
bottle of hoisin sauce, to serve

For the edamame and broccoli
150g Tenderstem broccoli
2 tablespoons untoasted
   sesame oil
120g frozen edamame beans
1 garlic clove, finely chopped
1 tablespoon finely grated
   fresh root ginger
1 tablespoon sesame seeds
salt

The vegan version of Peking duck! Aromatic, crispy shreds of jackfruit with plenty of hoisin sauce and crunchy cucumber. Jackfruit's main virtue is its texture, but it isn't a complete protein, so I've added a simple edamame bean side dish. I use untoasted sesame oil here, which you can buy in health food stores or online, rather than the more widely available toasted sesame oil, which is a flavour that tends to dominate.

Preheat the oven to 200°C (Gas Mark 6). Drain the jackfruit and break it up into coarse shreds. Mix it in a bowl with the soy sauce, five spice, vinegar, Szechuan pepper and sesame oil. Spread the mixture out on a baking tray and roast for 15–20 minutes, until starting to crisp and colour at the edges.

Meanwhile, halve the cucumber lengthways and remove and discard the seedy core with the tip of a teaspoon. Cut the rest into thin matchsticks. Trim the spring onions and shred them lengthways.

To make the edamame bean dish, boil or steam the broccoli for 3 minutes, until just tender. Heat the untoasted sesame oil in a wok or frying pan. Add the beans and broccoli and stir-fry for 2 minutes, until the beans have warmed through. Add the garlic, ginger, sesame seeds and a good pinch of salt. Cook for 1 more minute, making sure the garlic and ginger doesn't catch and burn.

When the jackfruit is ready, warm the pancakes. Take everything to the table so that people can build their own pancakes. Serve the beans and broccoli on the side.

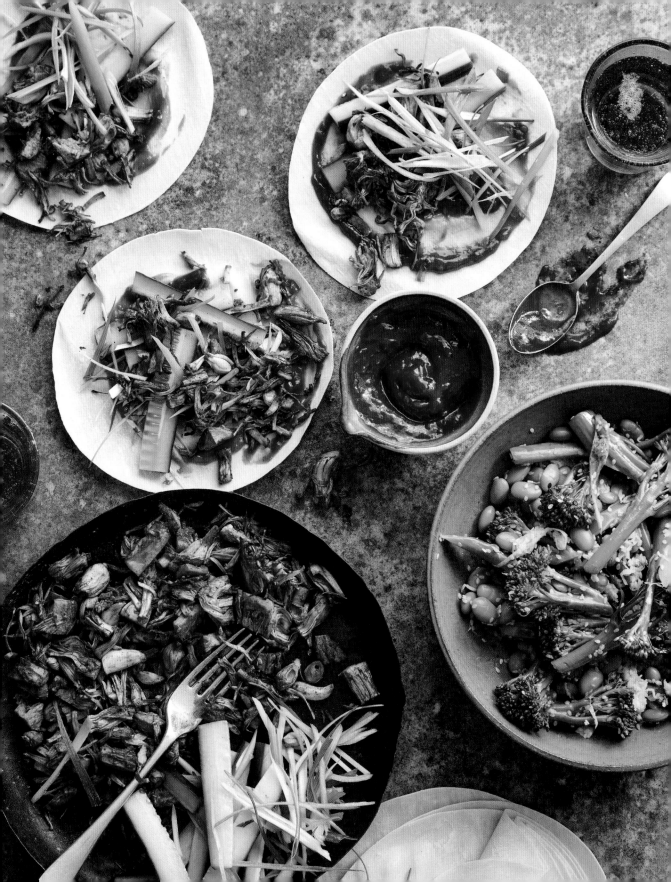

PIRI-PIRI TEMPEH TRAY BAKE WITH SWEET POTATO WEDGES

SERVES 2

200g tempeh
260g bottle piri-piri sauce
1 red pepper, deseeded
    and cut into 2cm chunks
1 yellow pepper, deseeded
    and cut into 2cm chunks
200g cherry tomatoes, halved
1 red onion, cut into wedges
4 tablespoons light olive oil
600g sweet potatoes
1 garlic clove, finely chopped
1 teaspoon thyme leaves
1 tablespoon red wine vinegar
lemon wedges, to serve
salt and pepper

Tempeh is tofu's whole-bean cousin, a more intense version made from fermented, pressed whole soy beans. Piri-piri is a readily available hot-and-sour sauce. Different brands pack varying punches, so use a little to marinate the tempeh and add more to taste at the end. I like to feel the chilli in my food, but you may not feel the same!

Preheat the oven to 200°C (Gas Mark 6). Cut the tempeh into 5mm-thick slices, then place it in a shallow bowl and mix it with 3 tablespoons of the piri-piri sauce. Set aside.

Throw the peppers, tomatoes and onion into a roasting tin with 2 tablespoons of oil and a generous seasoning of salt and pepper. Pop on the middle oven shelf for 10 minutes.

Meanwhile, cut the sweet potatoes into wedges, leaving the skin on. Place them in another roasting tin and toss them with the remaining oil and more salt and pepper. Pop them into the oven on the shelf above the veg and roast for 20–25 minutes, or until tender.

When the peppers have had 10 minutes, remove them from the oven and stir in the garlic, thyme and vinegar. Lay the marinated tempeh slices evenly on top, along with any sauce left in the bowl. Roast for a further 15 minutes, until the tempeh is nicely coloured.

Divide the sweet potato wedges between 2 warm plates and top with the roast veg and tempeh. Serve with lemon wedges and the rest of the piri-piri sauce, to pep things up to your required heat level.

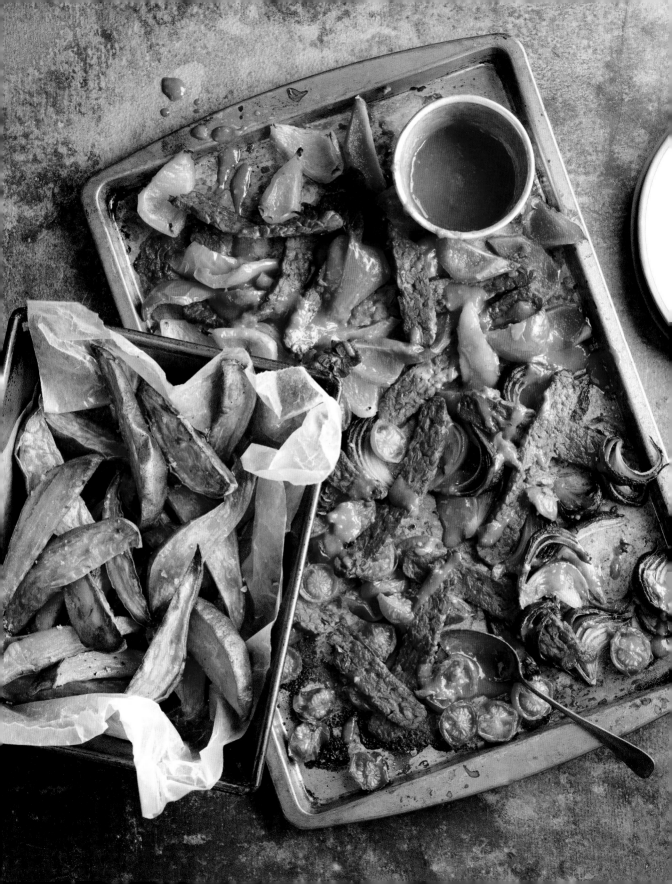

FAST and FURIOUS SOY and SRIRACHA STIR-FRY WITH RICE

SERVES 2

150g white basmati rice, rinsed
3 tablespoons vegetable oil
200g shiitake or oyster
    mushrooms, sliced
3 spring onions, sliced
1 courgette, sliced into ribbons
    with a vegetable peeler
100g sugar snap peas,
    trimmed and sliced
50g frozen peas
1 small head of pak choi, sliced
2cm piece of fresh root ginger,
    finely grated
2 garlic cloves, finely chopped
2 tablespoons soy sauce,
    or to taste
1 tablespoon sriracha sauce,
    or to taste
1 lime
leaves from a small bunch
    of coriander, chopped
30g salted cashew nuts,
    chopped
salt

The quantities of soy and sriracha here are a rough guide, as they're best added to taste. Armed with a bottle in each hand, you can tweak and fiddle like a mad scientist. Sriracha couldn't be hipper right now! You'll probably have more trouble sourcing the fresh veg than a bottle of the stuff. You can use whatever veg you have to hand, just make sure it is finely chopped and sliced so it cooks fast. Do all your prep before you start, as the cooking should be fast and furious.

Boil a kettle. Weigh the rice into a measuring jug and make a note of its volume, then tip it into a saucepan and cover with twice the volume of boiling water. Stir in a good pinch of salt, place over a medium-high heat and bring to the boil, then reduce the heat to a low simmer and cover. Cook for 10–12 minutes, until tender.

Heat 1 tablespoon of the oil in a wok or frying pan. Stir-fry the mushrooms over a high heat for 2 minutes, until cooked. Remove from the wok.

Heat the remaining 2 tablespoons of oil in the wok. Throw in the spring onions, courgette and sugar snap peas. Stir-fry over a high heat for 2 minutes, then return the mushrooms to the pan and add the peas, pak choi, ginger and garlic. Stir-fry for 1 more minute, until the leaves have wilted. Remove from the heat before adding the rice, soy and sriracha sauces and a good squeeze of lime juice. Mix well, taste and tweak with more soy, sriracha and lime juice until you're happy. Stir in the coriander, divide between warm bowls and sprinkle with the cashew nuts.

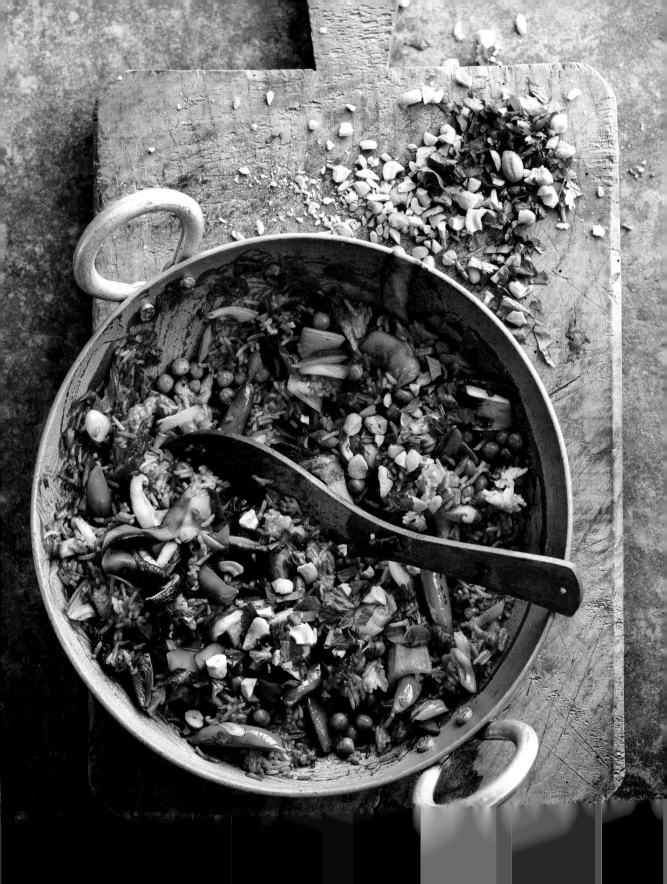

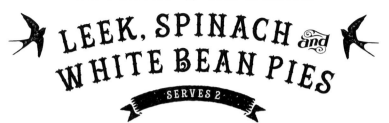

LEEK, SPINACH and WHITE BEAN PIES

SERVES 2

2 tablespoons olive oil,
  plus extra for the pastry
2 leeks, thinly sliced
1 garlic clove, finely chopped
1 teaspoon thyme leaves
1 tablespoon plain flour
200ml vegetable stock
  (see page 121 for homemade)
400g can cannellini beans,
  drained
150g baby spinach
1 lemon
pinch of ground nutmeg
6 filo pastry sheets
salt and pepper
150g Tenderstem broccoli,
  to serve

This couldn't be simpler. The filling just comes together in the pan and finishes cooking in the oven as the pastry colours. Don't be precious about the topping, just scrunch and tear the filo pastry sheets to give you lots of folds and edges that will crisp and colour – some might call it messy, but we'll say 'rustic'!

Preheat the oven to 180°C (Gas Mark 4). Warm the 2 tablespoons of olive oil in a saucepan. Fry the leeks gently with a pinch of salt for 5 minutes, until starting to soften.

Add the garlic, thyme and flour. Cook for 1 more minute, stirring well to stop the flour catching. Gradually stir in the stock, bit by bit, making sure there are no lumps.

Add the beans and spinach and warm them until the spinach has wilted; this will only take a couple of minutes. Remove from the heat and season with salt and pepper. Tweak with a squeeze or so of lemon juice and a pinch of nutmeg.

Transfer the bean mix into a snug pie dish, about 25 x 15cm. Brush each filo sheet lightly with olive oil, then roughly scrunch them on top of the pie and loosely tuck them in at the edges.

Transfer to the oven and bake for 25 minutes, or until the filo is golden and crisp.

When the pie is nearly ready, steam the broccoli for 3–4 minutes. Serve alongside the pie.

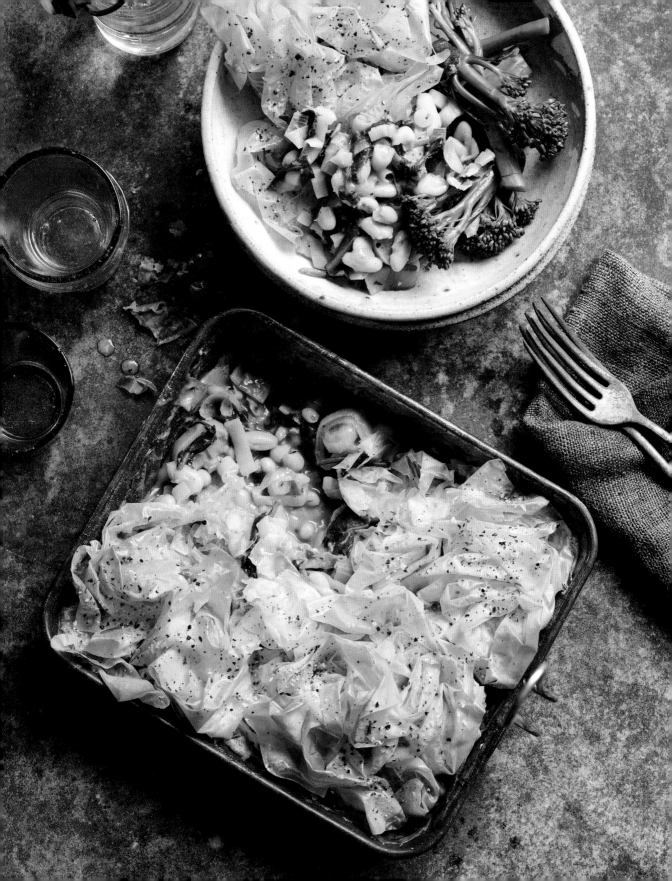

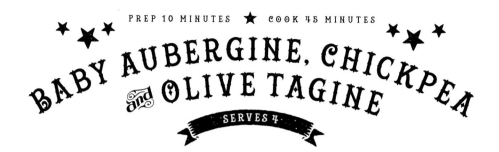

BABY AUBERGINE, CHICKPEA and OLIVE TAGINE

SERVES 4

800g baby aubergines, halved,
   or 2–3 regular aubergines,
   sliced into 1cm-thick slices
olive oil
1 large onion, sliced
2 small preserved lemons
3 garlic cloves, finely chopped
1 large tomato, roughly chopped
100g mixed olives, pitted
   and sliced
½ tablespoon ground ginger
½ tablespoon ground cumin
½ tablespoon ground coriander
1 teaspoon ground cinnamon
pinch of saffron threads
400g can chickpeas, including
   their liquid
400ml light vegetable stock
   (see page 121 for homemade)
250g couscous
leaves from a small bunch
   of coriander, chopped
leaves from a small bunch
   of parsley, chopped
salt

Aubergines like a bit of time to soften, but cook faster if you can get your hands on some of the baby varieties that are increasingly available. Preserved lemons are worth seeking out; their skin has a uniquely bitter, sour and salty taste.

Sprinkle the aubergine slices lighly with salt. Warm 2 tablespoons of olive oil in a large saucepan or casserole and cook the onion gently for 5 minutes, until starting to soften.

While the onion is cooking, cut open the lemons, scoop out and discard the pulpy insides and finely shred the skins. Add the garlic, tomato, olives, shredded preserved lemon and spices to the onion. Cook for 2 minutes, then add the chickpeas with all the liquid from the can. Pour in the stock, too, bring to the boil, then reduce the heat to a simmer. Pop a lid on and cook over a gentle heat for 15 minutes.

Boil a kettle. Put the couscous in a heatproof bowl and stir in 1 tablespoon of olive oil and a good pinch of salt. Pour over enough boiled water to cover the couscous by 2cm, then cover and leave to stand.

Heat a few tablespoons of olive oil in a frying pan and fry the aubergines, cut side down, for 3-4 minutes, until golden. You might need to do this in batches, adding more oil as you do. Add the aubergines to the tagine. Pop the lid back on and cook for another 20 minutes, until everything is tender. Taste and season if necessary, then stir in the herbs.

Fluff the couscous up with a fork to separate the grains and serve it alongside the tagine.

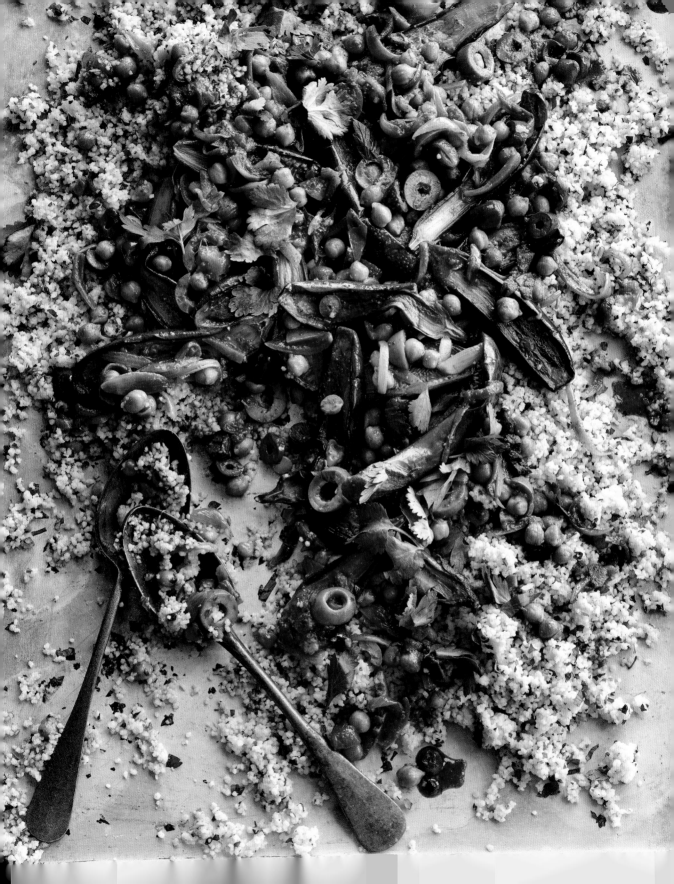

GUEST CHEF: PANCHO'S TACOS

SERVES 4

1 large cauliflower,
    cut into small florets
2 tablespoons olive oil
1 teaspoon chilli flakes
1 teaspoon ground cumin
1 teaspoon ground coriander
8 small soft tortillas, warmed
2 limes, cut into wedges,
    to serve

For the mango salsa
1 large red onion, finely diced
1–2 fresh chillies, finely
    chopped (depending
    on how hot you like it)
1 ripe mango, stone removed
    and cut into 1cm dice
250g canned sweetcorn,
    drained
large handful of fresh
    coriander leaves
zest of ½ lemon
juice of 1 lime

Ladies and Gents, let me introduce to you to my good friend Michael 'Pancho' Locke. He has kindly shared his taco recipe here – best served with a shedload of beers!

My first introduction to tacos was in Monterrey, Mexico. We were filming for the third series of Dirty Sanchez *and, after a long flight from Asia, we landed in Mexico exhausted and craving a good meal. We met with a Mexican fixer who promised he would take us to the best restaurant in Monterrey, which turned out to be a corrugated iron shack beside a petrol station in the middle of nowhere. Talk about looks can be deceiving! Simple layout, beers in buckets of ice, but the most delicious food with incredible salsas and condiments. Give these tacos a go – they're great for bringing everyone around the table for any occasion. They take me back to Monterrey every time!*

Preheat the oven to 200°C (Gas Mark 6). Put the cauliflower in a bowl, then add the olive oil and spices and toss to coat thoroughly. Place on to a baking tray and put those bad boys on the centre shelf of the oven for 25–30 minutes. Turn half way through so they cook evenly and are nicely browned.

Meanwhile make the salsa. Put the red onion, fresh chillies, mango, sweetcorn, coriander leaves, lemon zest and lime juice into a bowl. Season and mix well.

To assemble your tacos, place some of the spiced cauliflower filling in the centre of each warm tortilla. Top with the salsa, then fold each tortilla and eat with your fingers. Serve with lime wedges for squeezing over.

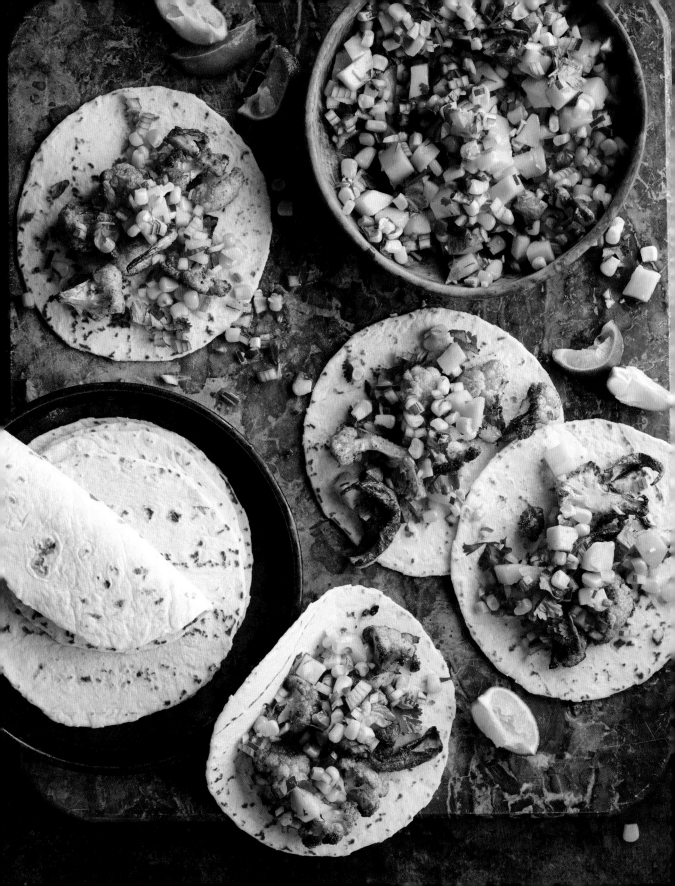

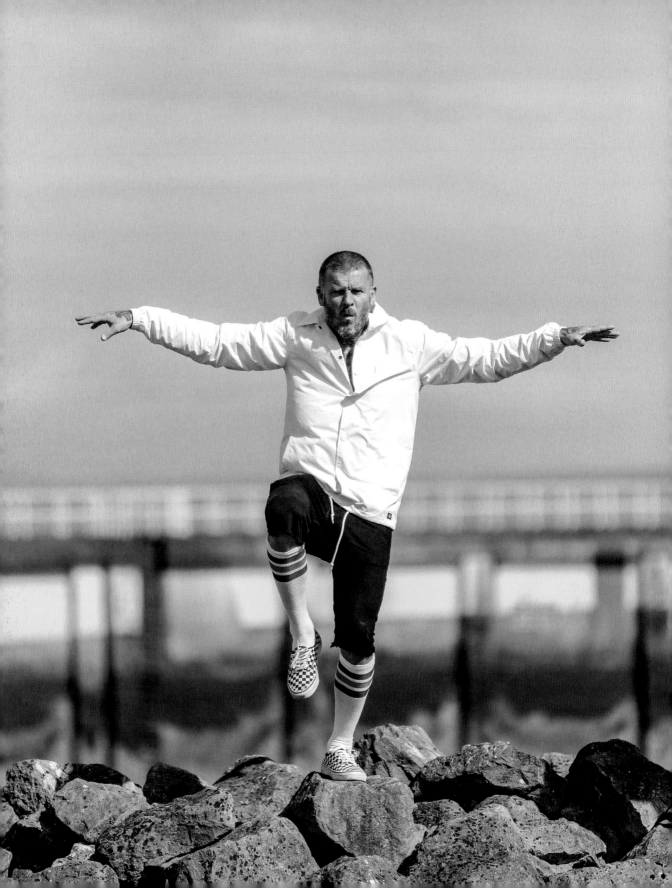

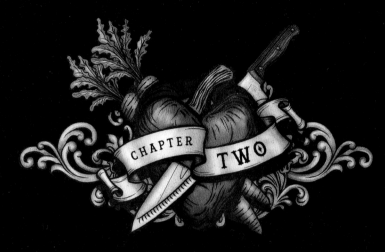

BALANCED

and

BANGING

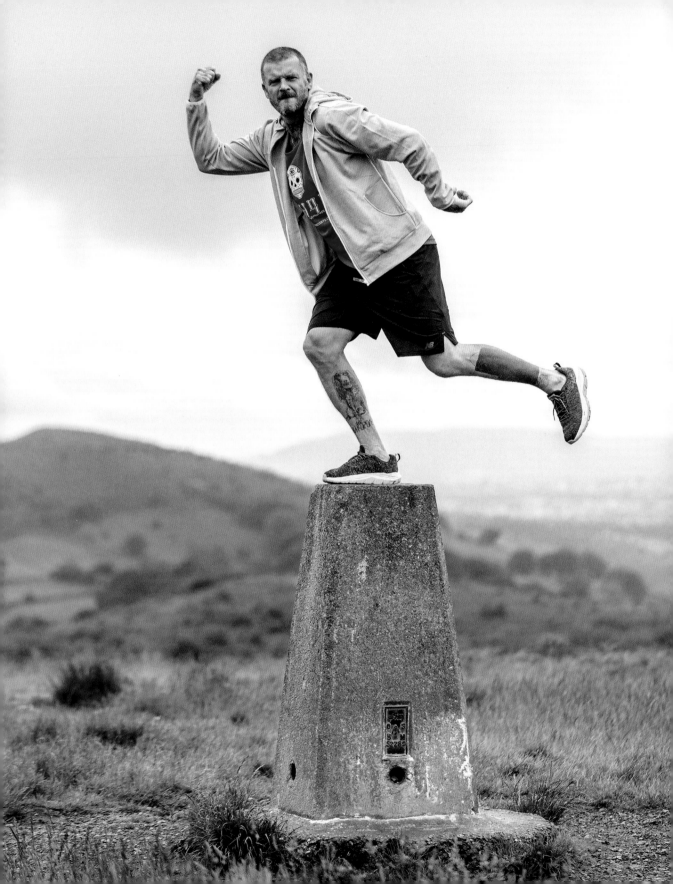

This may come as a surprise, but aside from when I was on *Dirty Sanchez* tours, I've always eaten well. I come from a generation in which you weren't allowed to be fussy: you ate what was put in front of you or you went without. Like many families, we didn't have much money, but my mother always made sure we had good food morning, noon and evening. She fed us healthy meals, packed with veg, that she cooked in the pressure cooker. That's a slightly touchy subject in my family ever since the first series of *Dirty Vegan* came out and I said on camera that my mother's veg was soggy as the pressure cooker always overcooked it!

Some days, my mam didn't have the money to feed us all; she would go without so that we children could eat. As we got older and more money started coming in, we would go shopping on a Saturday and visit the fruit and veg barrow on a side street outside the post office in Cardiff. Next we would go over to The Spice of Life – a health food store that sells nuts, seeds, pulses, spices, grains and so on – and buy Bombay mix for our Saturday nights in front of the TV, as we weren't allowed sweets. The Spice of Life still exists and I still shop there, visiting Gareth and his wife to get my health food supplies. It's one of my favourite food shops; it pre-dates the health food craze and still has unbeatable prices, as well as an amazing smell of spices in the air. And – of course – the greeting of Gareth's smile and his jokes that always make me laugh.

Even before becoming vegan I always loved veg. Veg is amazing and – when possible – organic is the way forward. The dishes in this chapter are a real celebration of the green stuff (and the red, yellow, orange, purple...) and are filling and flavour-packed, always with veg as the hero. Great for when you fancy a potter in the kitchen, exploring something new.

CAPONATA WITH BORLOTTI BEANS

SERVES 2 AS A MAIN OR 4 AS A SIDE

1 large aubergine,
  cut into 2cm cubes
5 tablespoons olive oil,
  plus extra if needed
1 red onion, sliced
3 celery sticks, finely chopped
1 courgette, cut into 1cm cubes
250g cherry tomatoes,
  roughly chopped
2 tablespoons tomato purée
2 tablespoon capers in brine,
  drained
60g pitted green olives,
  halved
40g sultanas
2 tablespoons red wine
  vinegar, or to taste
1 teaspoon light brown sugar
2 garlic cloves, finely chopped
pinch of chilli flakes, or to taste
400g can borlotti beans, drained
100ml water
leaves from 20g bunch of basil
30g flaked almonds, toasted
salt and pepper

A Sicilian dish that exemplifies the Italian principle of agrodolce (literally 'sour-sweet'). It is a stew of summer veg, not dissimilar to French ratatouille. The addition of beans isn't traditional, but makes it feel more like a complete meal.

Lightly salt the aubergine and leave it to sit for 10 minutes.

Heat 2 tablespoons of the olive oil in a deep frying pan or shallow casserole. Add the onion, celery and courgette and fry gently for 10 minutes, until the vegetables are starting to soften.

Add the tomatoes, tomato purée, capers, olives, sultanas, vinegar, sugar and garlic to the pan. Add the pinch of chilli flakes, season with salt and pepper, mix well and pop on a lid. Leave over a gentle heat while you fry the aubergine.

Place a separate frying pan over a high heat and add the remaining 3 tablespoons of olive oil. Fry the aubergine for 4–5 minutes, until golden. You may need to do this in batches, adding more oil if you do so.

Add the aubergines and beans to the pan along with the measured water. Pop the lid back on and cook very gently for 20 minutes, until everything is tender.

Taste and tweak with some more salt, pepper, vinegar and chilli to taste. Tear in the basil and serve with the almonds scattered over the top.

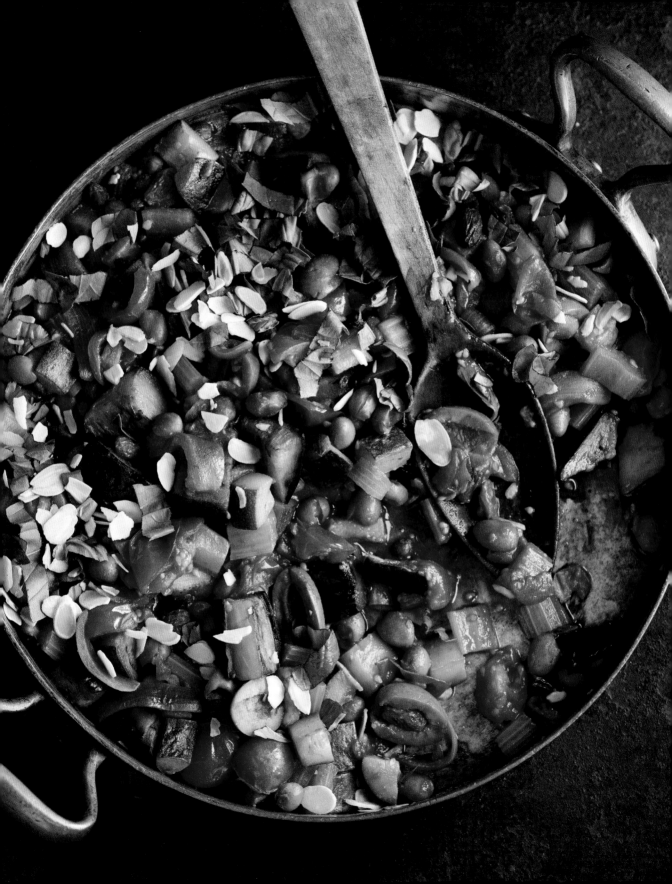

SCANDI BEETROOT, POTATO and FENNEL SALAD

SERVES 2

400g small summer beetroots
½ teaspoon caraway seeds
finely grated zest and juice
    of 1 orange
2 tablespoons olive oil
300g waxy new potatoes
1 small fennel bulb, thinly sliced
100g radishes, cut into wedges
    and slices
½ small red onion,
    very thinly sliced
1 tablespoon freshly grated
    horseradish
1 tablespoon red wine vinegar
2 tablespoons vegan
    crème fraîche
50g watercress, any coarse
    stalks removed
bunch of dill, any coarse stalks
    removed, finely chopped
salt and pepper
dark rye bread, to serve

There's no need to make a separate dressing for this dish, as the liquid left in the roasting tin is almost enough and is easily built on. Serve the lot warm, or leave everything to cool before folding in the watercress. I recommend adding a bit of vegan crème fraîche – there are some much better products on the market than there were a few years ago, but I'd recommend avoiding anything that tastes or smells strongly of coconut.

Preheat the oven to 200°C (Gas Mark 6). Peel the beetroots and cut them into wedges. Place them in a small roasting tin with the caraway, half the orange juice, the olive oil and plenty of salt and pepper. Mix well, cover with foil and roast for about 40 minutes, or until tender.

Meanwhile, put the potatoes into a pan of cold salted water. Bring to the boil and cook for 10–12 minutes, or until cooked through, then drain. When they are cool enough to handle, slice them into thick discs.

When the beets are ready, add the potatoes, fennel, radishes and onion to the pan, along with the horseradish and vinegar. Mix well and adjust the seasoning to your liking. Just before serving, fold in the crème fraîche (if using) and watercress. Taste and add a little more orange juice, if you think it needs it.

Pile on to plates and garnish with the dill and a sprinkle of orange zest. Serve with slices of rye bread on the side.

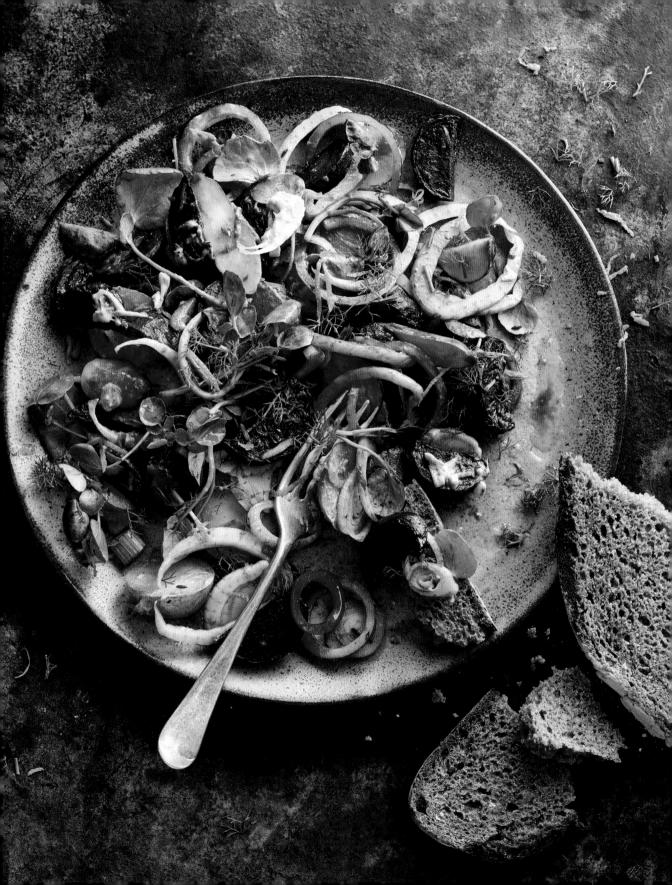

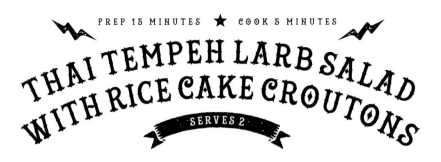

THAI TEMPEH LARB SALAD WITH RICE CAKE CROUTONS

SERVES 2

300g tempeh
2 tablespoons vegetable oil
3 wholegrain rice cakes
leaves from a small bunch
    of basil, chopped
leaves from a small bunch
    of mint, chopped
leaves from a small bunch
    of coriander, chopped
40g salted peanuts,
    roughly chopped
1 Little Gem lettuce,
    leaves separated
2 spring onions, thinly sliced
½ cucumber, sliced into ribbons
    with a vegetable peeler
4–6 radishes, thinly sliced

For the dressing
1 shallot or ½ small red onion,
    finely chopped
½ tablespoon chilli flakes
    (ideally Thai), or to taste
juice of 2 limes
2 tablespoons tamari
    or soy sauce
1 lemon grass stalk, pale bulb
    end only, peeled and
    roughly chopped
2 lime leaves, thinly sliced
    (optional)
½ tablespoon brown sugar
salt

To serve
lime wedges
rice (optional)

This dish is traditionally made with minced meat, so tempeh is an ace substitute as it can be chopped down into a similar texture, is full of protein and will carry the punchy dressing well. An important part of a larb is toasted and ground rice, but making that can add a good 20 minutes to the prep time, so I've opted for a timesaver by crumbling in a couple of rice cakes instead. (I tried toasting the rice cakes first to see if it added to their flavour; it turns out they are quite dangerously flammable – I nearly lost my eyebrows. A no-no for the toaster, but ideal as emergency tinder.)

Put all the dressing ingredients into a small food processor and blitz into a paste. It wants to be hot, sharp and salty, so add more chilli or a pinch more salt if you think it needs it.

Chop the tempeh until it has the texture of mince. Heat the oil in a wok or frying pan until it is very hot. Add the tempeh and stir-fry for 2–3 minutes, until golden and cooked through. Remove from the heat and stir in the dressing. Leave for 5 minutes, to let everything get to know each other.

Break the rice cakes into small crouton-like pieces and fold them into the tempeh, along with the herbs and peanuts. Taste and tweak with more salt, if you think it needs it.

Serve alongside the lettuce and veg, with lime wedges on the side. The best way to eat it is to scoop some tempeh on to a lettuce leaf, top it with plenty of sliced veg and a good squeeze of lime juice. You can serve it with some freshly cooked rice, if you want a more substantial meal.

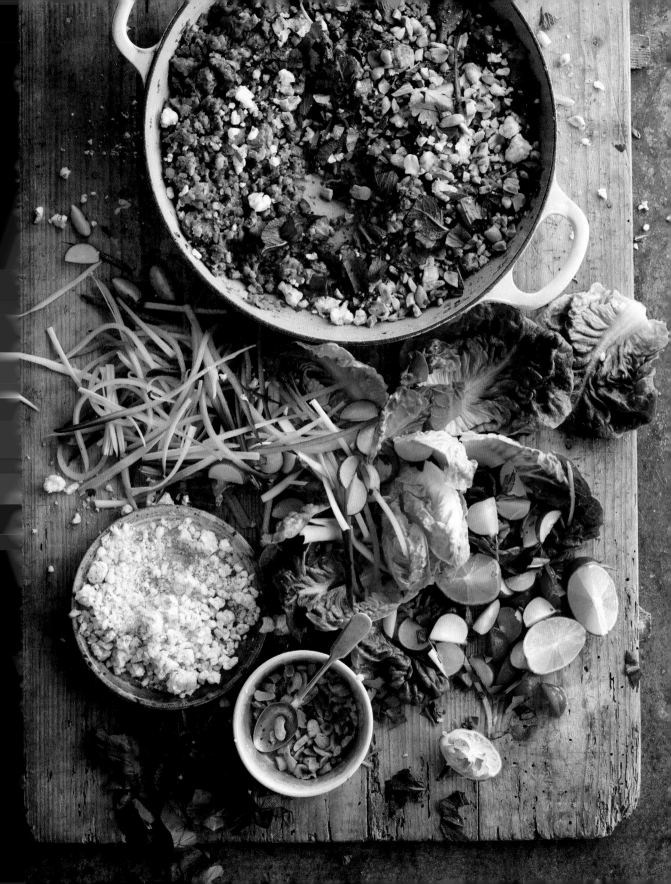

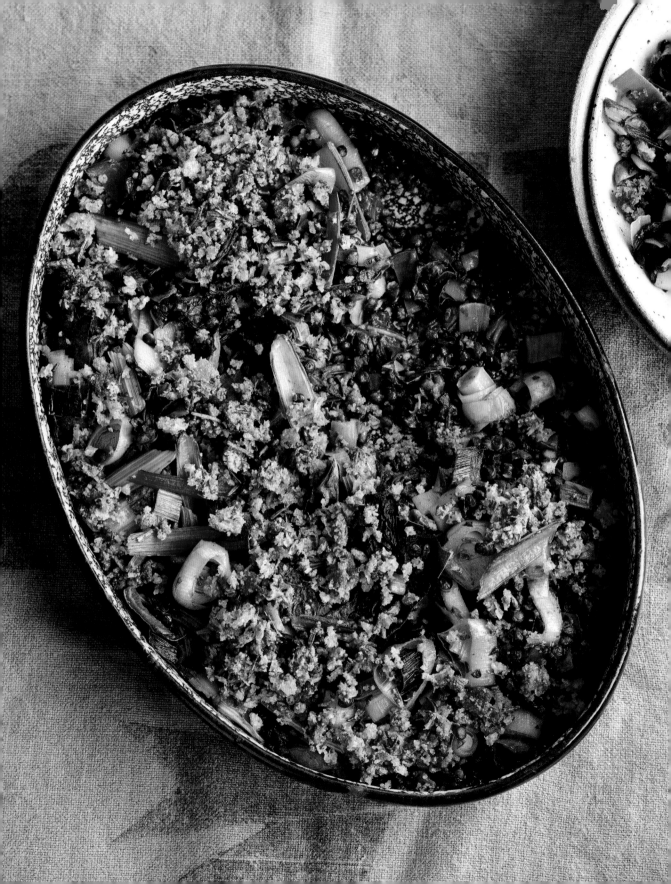

RAINBOW CHARD, LEEK and LENTIL GRATIN

SERVES 2

300g rainbow chard
3 tablespoons olive oil
2 large leeks, sliced
2 garlic cloves, finely chopped
2 bay leaves
400g can Puy lentils, drained
125ml white wine
300ml vegetable stock
   (see page 121 for homemade)
½ tablespoon wholegrain
   mustard
200g stale sourdough bread
½ tablespoon chopped
   rosemary leaves
finely grated zest of
   1 unwaxed lemon
salt and pepper

You can, of course, make this with regular green Swiss chard, but it seems so much cheerier with some brightly coloured stalks in the mix. It is pretty much a meal in itself, but you can take it to another level if you serve it with some roast potatoes or fat wedges of roast squash on the side. If you want to make it a bit richer, stir in a few tablespoons of vegan crème fraîche.

Preheat the oven to 180°C (Gas Mark 4). Split the chard stalks away from the leaves. Roughly slice the stalks and set the leaves aside.

Heat 2 tablespoons of the olive oil in a saucepan and gently sweat the chard and leeks with a pinch of salt for 10 minutes, until softened.

Add the garlic and bay leaves and cook for 2 more minutes before adding the lentils and wine. Let it bubble away until the liquid has disappeared into the lentils. Tip in the stock, bring to the boil, then reduce the heat to a simmer and stir in the chard leaves until they have just wilted. Remove from the heat, stir in the mustard and season well to taste.

Remove and discard the crusts from the bread, then tear it into chunks and place it into a food processor with the rosemary, lemon zest and the remaining 1 tablespoon of olive oil. Blitz into coarse crumbs.

Pack the lentil mixture into a snug gratin dish. Cover with an even layer of breadcrumbs and bake for 20 minutes, until the crumbs are golden and crisp.

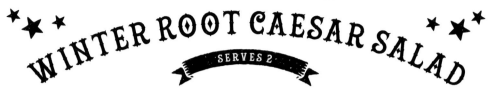

WINTER ROOT CAESAR SALAD

SERVES 2

400g parsnips, cut into
  chunky batons
400g carrots, cut into
  chunky batons
4 shallots, cut into wedges
olive oil
2 thick slices of sourdough
  bread, crusts removed
  and bread torn into
  bite-sized pieces
1 tablespoon capers
  in brine, drained
150g curly kale, stalks
  removed, leaves torn
  into bite-sized pieces
handful of radicchio
  or chicory leaves
salt and pepper

For the dressing
50g blanched almonds,
  soaked in water overnight,
  then drained
1 garlic clove, finely grated
½ tablespoon Dijon mustard
1 tablespoon brine from
  the caper jar
2 tablespoons lemon juice
2 tablespoons nutritional yeast
2 tablespoons olive oil
3 tablespoons boiling water

A proper tasty salad. Both kale and radicchio leaves are bitter, so the dressing here needs to be strong: creamy, garlicky and sharp all at the same time.

Preheat the oven to 200°C (Gas Mark 6). Place the carrots and parsnips in a large roasting tray with the shallots. Oil and season them all well and roast for 25–30 minutes, until tender. Set aside to cool slightly.

Meanwhile, place the bread pieces on a baking sheet and mix with 2 tablespoons of oil and a good pinch of salt, turning them well. Pop them in the oven alongside the carrots for 12–15 minutes, turning once or twice, until golden and crisp.

To make the dressing, place all the ingredients in a food processor. Blend until smooth, stopping to scrape down the sides every so often. It should be thick with the consistency of yogurt. Taste and tweak the seasoning.

Heat a few tablespoons of oil in a small frying pan. Fry the capers for 2–3 minutes, until they start to open and turn crisp at the edges. Remove to a piece of kitchen paper to soak up the oil and leave to cool.

Place the kale in a mixing bowl with a pinch of salt and a small dash of oil. Massage the leaves for a few minutes by scrunching them with your hands; this works the salt into the leaves and helps to tenderize them.

Add the radicchio to the kale along with the parsnips, carrots, shallots, croutons and 2 tablespoons of the dressing. Mix well and divide between 2 plates. Spoon over the rest of the dressing and garnish with the crispy capers.

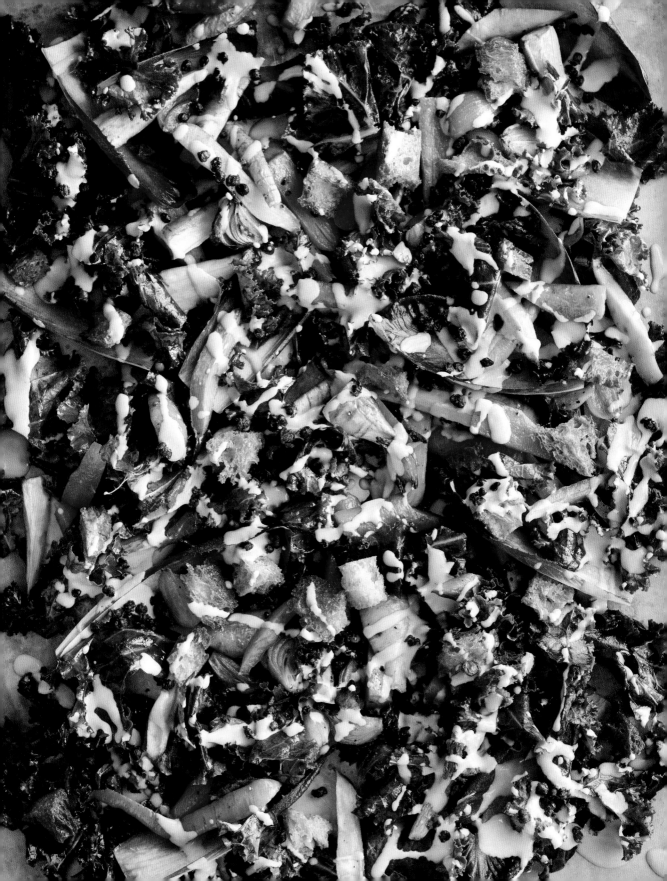

JERK STEW WITH ACKEE

SERVES 2

For the stew
2 tablespoons vegetable oil
3 spring onions, sliced
400g sweet potatoes,
    cut into 2cm cubes
1 garlic clove, finely chopped
2 tablespoons jerk seasoning
    (see below)
400g can chopped tomatoes
400g can black-eyed beans,
    drained
400ml vegetable stock
    (see page 121 for homemade)
100g baby spinach
1 lime
1 tablespoon peanut butter
    (optional)
salt and pepper

For the ackee
1 tablespoon vegetable oil
2 spring onions, sliced
150g roasted peppers, sliced
540g can ackee, drained

For the jerk seasoning
1 tablespoon allspice berries
1 tablespoon black peppercorns
1 tablespoon dried thyme
½ tablespoon caster sugar
1 teaspoon cayenne pepper
1 teaspoon ground cinnamon
½ teaspoon ground ginger
½ teaspoon ground nutmeg

Ackee is a tropical fruit with soft, creamy flesh. It is often used in vegan cooking as a scrambled egg substitute, as it resembles them both in appearance and texture. Canned ackee is sold in larger supermarkets or online. If it isn't to your taste, just serve the stew with rice instead. The addition of peanut butter is inspired by a pub snack of jerk-spiced peanuts that stuck in the mind...

To make the jerk seasoning, grind everything together in a mortar and pestle, blender or spice grinder. Store in an airtight jar until needed.

Now make the stew. Warm the oil in a saucepan. Add the spring onions, sweet potatoes and a pinch of salt. Cook gently for 5 minutes, until the spring onions start to soften. Add the garlic and jerk seasoning to the pan and cook for 1 minute, stirring to make sure the spices don't burn. Tip in the tomatoes, beans and stock. Bring to the boil, then reduce the heat to a simmer and cook for 20 minutes, until the sweet potatoes are tender. Mix the peanut butter, if using, with a ladle of liquid and add to the pan.

Meanwhile, cook the ackee. Warm the oil in a frying pan. Add the spring onions and fry them over a medium heat for 5 minutes, until softened. Add the peppers and the ackee. Cook for 5 minutes, stirring very gently every so often, until warmed through.

When the stew is ready, stir in the spinach until wilted. Taste and tweak the seasoning with salt, pepper and a squeeze or so of lime juice. Serve the ackee alongside the stew, as you would rice.

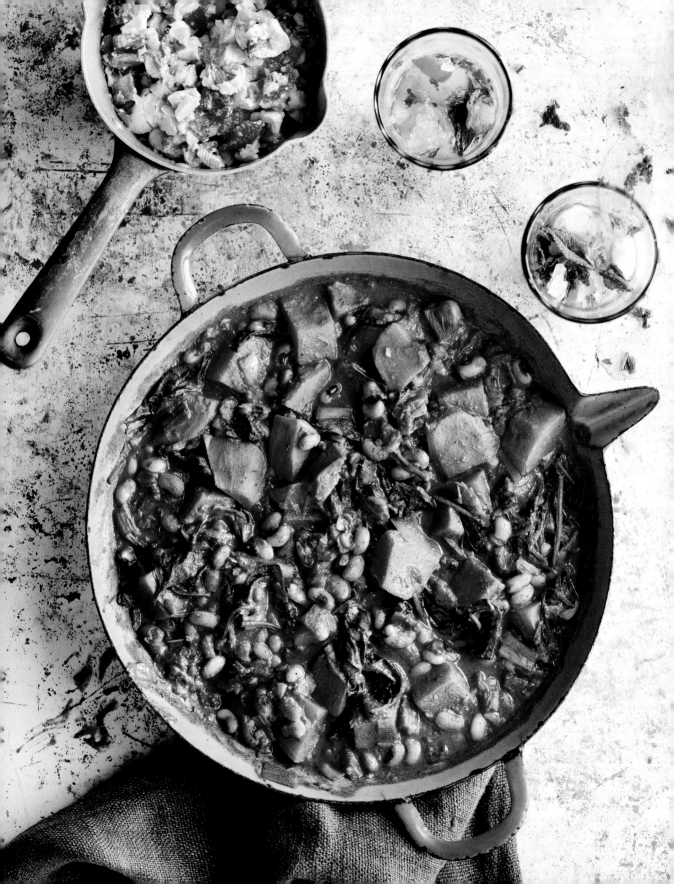

MINTY COURGETTES WITH POPPED BEANS and TAHINI

SERVES 2

2 courgettes, cut into rough
   3cm angular pieces
400g asparagus spears,
   woody ends snapped off
4 tablespoons extra virgin
   olive oil
finely grated zest and juice
   of 1 unwaxed lemon
handful of mint leaves, shredded
400g can butter beans
   or cannellini beans,
   drained and rinsed
½ teaspoon fennel seeds
salt and pepper

For the sauce
4 tablespoons light tahini
juice of ½ lemon
2 teaspoons light soy sauce
1 teaspoon maple syrup
   or agave syrup
3–6 tablespoons water

This pile of herby, smoky green vegetables is a proper riot of summer flavours (even when it's raining), and 'popping' the canned beans in the oven in this way makes a nice change. Using a griddle pan makes the charred vegetables look really tempting on the plate but, if you don't have one, cook them under the grill instead. This is delicious with couscous, or spooned on top of flatbreads, for a more substantial meal.

Preheat the oven to 220°C (Gas Mark 7). Heat a griddle pan over a high heat for at least 5 minutes until smoking hot. Cook the courgettes and asparagus spears – in batches to prevent overcrowding – for 4–5 minutes each side, until deep char marks form. Toss the vegetables in a bowl with the olive oil, lemon zest and juice and mint leaves, then season well with salt and pepper. Allow the flavours to muddle while the vegetables are warm.

Dry the beans on a plate lined with kitchen paper, then toss them into a shallow roasting tin with the fennel seeds. Place on the middle shelf of the oven for 18–20 minutes, until the beans split and pop and are colouring in places.

Mix all the ingredients except the water together for the sauce, then loosen with the water, adding it gradually, until the sauce has the consistency of thin yogurt.

Arrange the vegetables on a plate with the lemony, minty dressing from the bowl, scatter over the popped beans and drizzle over a spoonful of the sauce, keeping a bit back for spooning over the vegetables at the table.

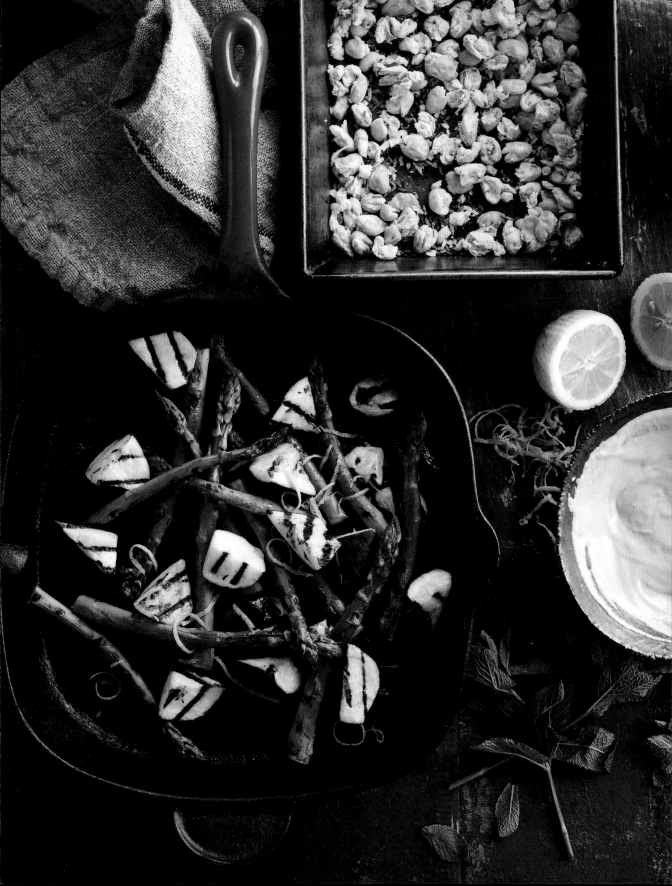

STUFFED COURGETTE FLOWERS WITH TOMATOES and FARRO

SERVES 2

For the flowers

2 tablespoons olive oil
2 courgettes, grated
1 garlic clove, finely chopped
1 tablespoon capers in brine,
    drained and chopped
30g pine nuts, roughly chopped
leaves from a small bunch
    of basil, chopped
leaves from a small bunch
    of parsley, chopped
1 unwaxed lemon
6 large courgette flowers
salt and pepper
good crusty bread, to serve

For the sauce

2 tablespoons olive oil
1 red onion, sliced
2 garlic cloves, finely chopped
175ml white wine
400g tomatoes, roughly chopped
40g pitted black olives, sliced
50g farro
1 bay leaf
400ml light vegetable stock
    (see page 121 for homemade)

Courgette flowers might be difficult to come by in the shops, but if you know someone with an allotment or even a passing interest in growing veg, chances are they'll have them in abundance come midsummer. You can pinch some of their courgettes for the filling and – if you are lucky – you may even be able to pilfer some tomatoes and basil, too. Get to know a gardener!

To start the filling for the courgette flowers, warm the olive oil in a saucepan. Add the courgettes and a pinch of salt. Cook them very gently for 15 minutes, stirring often, until softened and collapsed. When cooked, remove them from the heat to cool for a bit.

Meanwhile, start the sauce. Warm the olive oil in a wide-based saucepan or casserole. Add the red onion and a pinch of salt. Cook gently for 10 minutes, until starting to soften. Add the garlic and wine and cook for 2 minutes, until the wine has reduced by half, then add the tomatoes, olives, farro, bay leaf and stock. Bring to the boil, then reduce the heat to a simmer and pop on the lid. Cook gently for 15 minutes.

Meanwhile, to finish the filling, stir the garlic, capers, pine nuts and herbs into the courgettes. Finely zest half the lemon and add that, too, then season with salt and pepper. Gently open the courgette flowers and cut away and discard the stamen inside. Gently wash them, to get rid of any bugs. Carefully place a generous spoonful of the filling into the centre of each flower and fold the petals back together to close them up again.

When the tomato sauce has had 15 minutes, taste and tweak the seasoning with salt and pepper, adding a dash more water if it looks a little too dry. It wants to be fairly loose, as the courgette flowers need liquid to braise in.

Place the courgette flowers into the pan, pop the lid back on, and cook over a low heat for a final 15 minutes, until the flowers and filling are cooked through and the farro is tender. Fish out the bay leaf, if you can find it.

Serve with the remaining lemon, cut into wedges, and plenty of crusty bread to soak up the winey sauce.

BAKED SQUASH SPELTOTTO

SERVES 4–6

1 butternut squash, peeled,
　deseeded and cut into
　2cm chunks (about 700g
　prepared weight)
4 garlic cloves
½ small bunch of thyme,
　woody stalks removed
olive oil
1 tablespoon wholegrain mustard
1 tablespoon brown miso
1 large onion, finely chopped
½ teaspoon chilli flakes
½ teaspoon ground cinnamon
250g pearled spelt
125ml dry sherry or dry
　white wine
1 litre vegetable stock
　(for homemade, see page 121)
150g kale, roughly chopped
50g hazelnuts, toasted
　and chopped
salt and pepper

Whizzed up with garlic cloves, the caramalized roast squash forms a deeply flavoured, creamy sauce for this baked spelt risotto. Unlike traditional risottos, there's no standing and constant stirring needed with this recipe.

Preheat the oven to 200°C (Gas Mark 6). Toss the butternut squash in a deep roasting tin with the garlic, thyme and enough olive oil to coat. Season well. Place in the hot oven for 30 minutes, or until the squash is soft throughout and beginning to catch at the edges. Leave the oven on.

Put three-quarters of the roasted squash into a food processor with the thyme. When the garlic cloves are cool enough to handle, squeeze them from their skins and add them to the processor too, along with the mustard and miso. Blitz on a high speed until smooth.

Heat 3 tablespoons of olive oil in a large ovenproof sauté pan (about 28cm) over a medium heat. Cook the onion with a pinch of salt for about 8 minutes, or until soft and translucent. Stir in the chilli and cinnamon and cook for a minute until the spices smell fragrant. Add the spelt and stir for a minute so the oil and spices coat every grain. Pour in the sherry or wine and stir until it has been completely absorbed. Add the blitzed squash, stock and kale and bring to the boil. Stir through the roasted squash and hazelnuts and carefully place on a shelf at the top of the oven.

Bake for 45 minutes, opening the oven door 2–3 times during the cooking time to release some steam and check that the top of the speltotto isn't burning. If it looks as though it's catching, cover with foil until the timer pings.

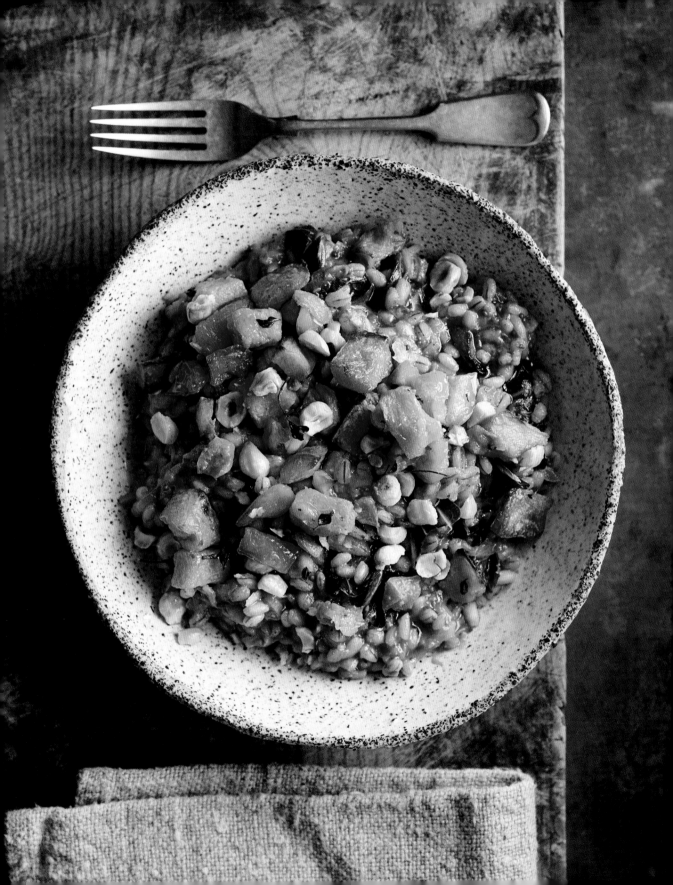

⚡ SATAY BROCCOLI ⚡ WITH CRISPY ONIONS

SERVES 4 AS A SIDE OR 2 AS A MAIN

For the satay sauce
4 tablespoons peanut butter
 (smooth and crunchy
 both work well)
1 shallot, finely chopped
1 garlic clove, finely chopped
1 tablespoon light soy sauce,
 or to taste
1 teaspoon rice wine vinegar
1 teaspoon agave syrup or light
 brown sugar, or to taste
juice of 1 lime, or to taste
¼ teaspoon chilli flakes

For the broccoli
1 large head of broccoli, broken
 into bite-sized florets, stalks
 roughly peeled and cut into
 2cm cubes
2 tablespoons toasted sesame oil

For the crispy onions
300ml vegetable or sunflower oil
1 onion, thinly sliced on a
 mandolin or with a sharp knife
100g cornflour
sea salt flakes

Peanuts and broccoli work so well together. Make sure you use the broccoli stalk too; it's nuts that we've been taught to chuck it! With a bit of love, it's as tasty as the rest. You can use shop-bought crispy onions – find them in most large supermarkets as well as Indian and Thai supermarkets.

Preheat the oven to 220°C (Gas Mark 7). Make the satay sauce first by mixing all the ingredients together. Loosen with enough water to give the mixture the consistency of thick pouring cream. Taste and tweak. Set aside.

Toss the broccoli with the sesame oil in a shallow roasting tin in a single layer, then place in the oven for 10 minutes. Remove from the oven and spoon over half the satay sauce, using a spatula to make sure every piece of broccoli is covered, and return to the oven for a final 10 minutes, until beginning to catch and blacken at the edges.

Meanwhile, heat the vegetable oil in a wide frying pan over a medium heat. Toss the sliced onion in a bowl with the cornflour until every piece is entirely coated. Test the heat of the oil by dropping a piece of onion into the pan. If it bubbles and turns golden in 15 seconds, the oil is ready. Fry the onion in 2–3 batches, lifting each batch out when golden with a slotted spoon on to a plate lined with kitchen paper. Sprinkle the onion with sea salt flakes after it has been out of the pan for a couple of minutes.

Remove the broccoli from the oven and drizzle with the remaining satay sauce. Serve with the crispy onions on top.

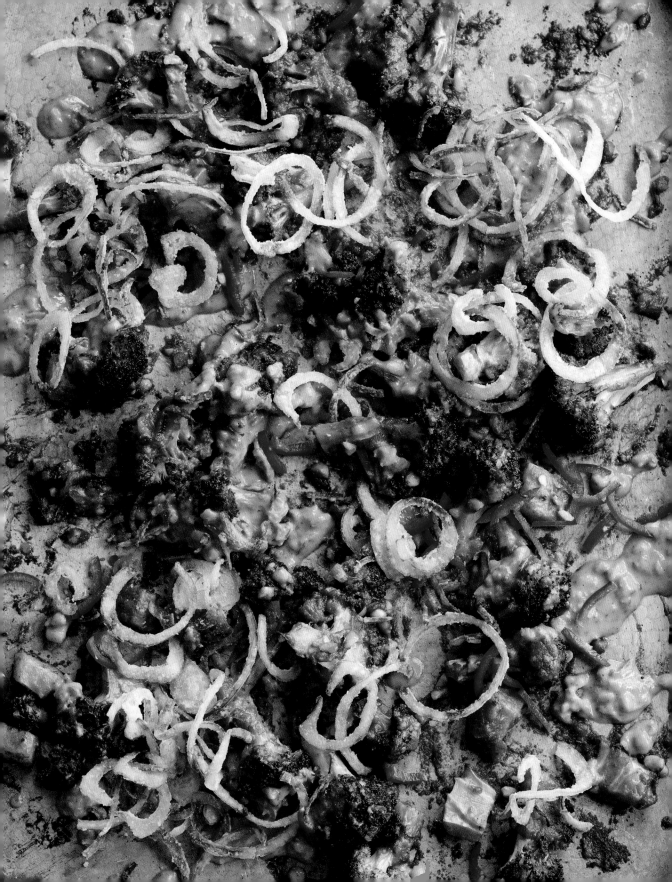

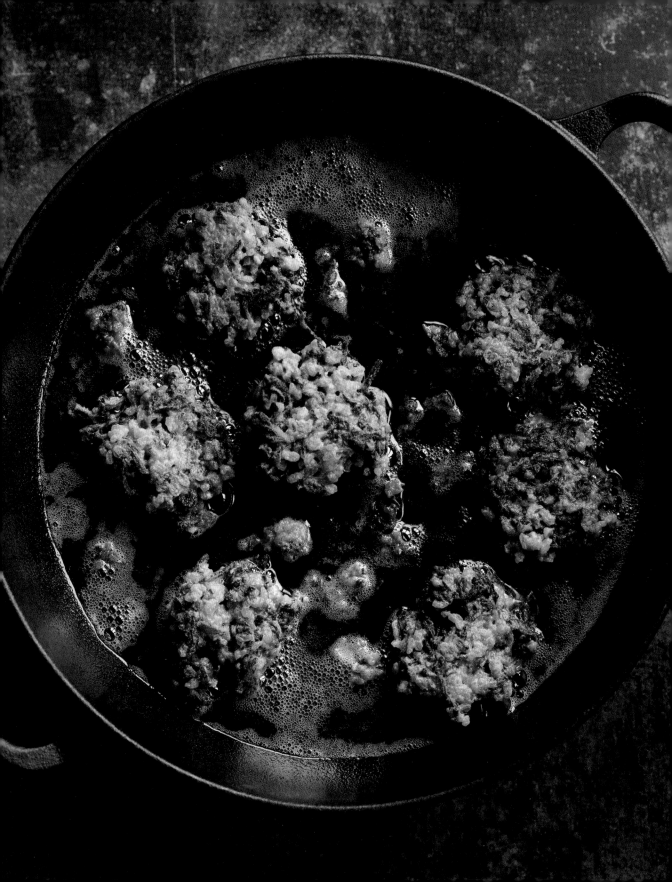

FREEKEH STINGER FRITTERS

SERVES 2 AS A MAIN OR 4 AS A SNACK

For the fritters
60g gram (chickpea) flour
1 tablespoon olive oil
90ml water
60g cracked freekeh
100g young stinging nettle tops
1 unwaxed lemon
1 teaspoon ground cumin
1 garlic clove, finely chopped
vegetable oil, for frying
salt and pepper

For the vegetables
2 tablespoons olive oil
150g asparagus, trimmed
    and cut into 3cm pieces
1 Little Gem lettuce,
    cut into 8 wedges
3 spring onions, sliced
100g peas, fresh or frozen
leaves from a small bunch
    of parsley, chopped
6 large mint leaves, chopped
vegan mayonnaise or chilli
    sauce, to serve (optional)

These are based on the freaky freekeh pancakes I made in the first TV series, with a simple chickpea flour batter fortified with nutty, ancient grains. The best time for picking stinging nettles is in the spring, as it is the young tender leaves that you want to harvest. Take a pair of rubber gloves for picking, unless you feel the need to suffer for your art. Nettles grow abundantly and are easily identified, so it will take you no time to fill a bag. Wild garlic carpets the woods at this time of year too and can be used as a less perilous substitute, though make sure you pick carefully! You can also just use some spinach in the same way.

Put a kettle on to boil. Preheat the oven to 150°C (Gas Mark 2). While you wait, whisk the gram flour together with the olive oil and measured cold water in a large mixing bowl. Set aside.

Put the freekeh in a saucepan and cover with 200ml of boiling water. Add a generous pinch of salt and bring to the boil, then reduce the heat to a gentle simmer. Cook for 15 minutes, or until the grains are tender and most of the water has evaporated.

While the freekeh cooks, place the nettle tops in a bowl. Cover with boiling water and let them sit for 1 minute, or a few moments more, until visibly wilted. Drain, return to the bowl and cool under cold water immediately. Drain again and squeeze out any excess water: you can use your bare hands now, as the hot water disarms the stings. Roughly chop the leaves.

Recipe continues overleaf

Drain any water away from the cooked freekeh and tip it into the bowl with the batter. Finely zest half the lemon and add that too, followed by the nettle tops, cumin and garlic. Season with salt and pepper to taste.

Add a shallow layer of oil to a frying pan over a medium-high heat. Dollop heaped dessertspoons of the fritter mix into the pan and flatten them out with the back of a spoon. Fry for 2–3 minutes on each side, until golden, in batches of no more than 6 at a time. You should get 10–12 fritters from the mix. Slide them all on to a baking tray and pop them in the oven for 10 minutes while you cook the veg.

Wipe clean the frying pan you cooked the fritters in. Add the olive oil and place over a medium-high heat. Add the asparagus and lettuce with a pinch of salt. Sauté them for 3–4 minutes, until lightly colouring. Add the spring onions and peas and cook for another 2–3 minutes, keeping it all moving, until everything is tender. Finish with a good squeeze of lemon juice, season with salt and pepper and mix in the herbs.

Serve the veg with the fritters, with your dipping sauce of choice.

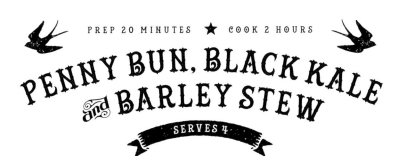

PENNY BUN, BLACK KALE and BARLEY STEW

SERVES 4

750g penny bun mushrooms
olive oil
2 onions, sliced
3 celery sticks, finely chopped
2 carrots, finely chopped
3 garlic cloves, finely chopped
1 teaspoon chopped
    rosemary leaves
1 teaspoon chopped
    thyme leaves
2 bay leaves
125g pearled barley
175ml white wine
800ml vegetable stock,
    preferably dark and with
    mushrooms (see page 121)
150g black kale
leaves from a small bunch
    of parsley, chopped
salt

'Penny bun' is the old British name for the mushroom now more commonly known as cep or porcini. It is worth seeking out, as both the taste and texture are amazing, though you'll have to save this recipe for late summer and early autumn. Serve with celeriac mash for an even heartier dish.

Preheat the oven to 150°C (Gas Mark 2). Halve or quarter the mushrooms, depending on their size. Heat 2 tablespoons of olive oil in a large saucepan or casserole. Fry the mushrooms with a pinch of salt over a high heat for 3–4 minutes, until lightly coloured but by no means completely cooked. Remove from the pan.

Add some more oil and gently sweat the onions, celery and carrots for 10 minutes, until starting to soften. Add the garlic, herbs and barley and cook for 3 more minutes. Tip in the wine and let it cook until it has been absorbed by the barley, then pour in the stock, return the mushrooms and bring to the boil. Reduce the heat to a simmer and season well. Put on a lid and transfer it to the oven

Meanwhile, strip away and discard the kale stalks and roughly shred the leaves. After the stew has cooked for 40 minutes, stir the kale into the pan and return it to the oven for a final 30 minutes (black kale can handle a long cook). When ready, taste and tweak the seasoning and remove the bay leaves if you can find them.

Serve the stew in shallow warm bowls, sprinkled with chopped parsley.

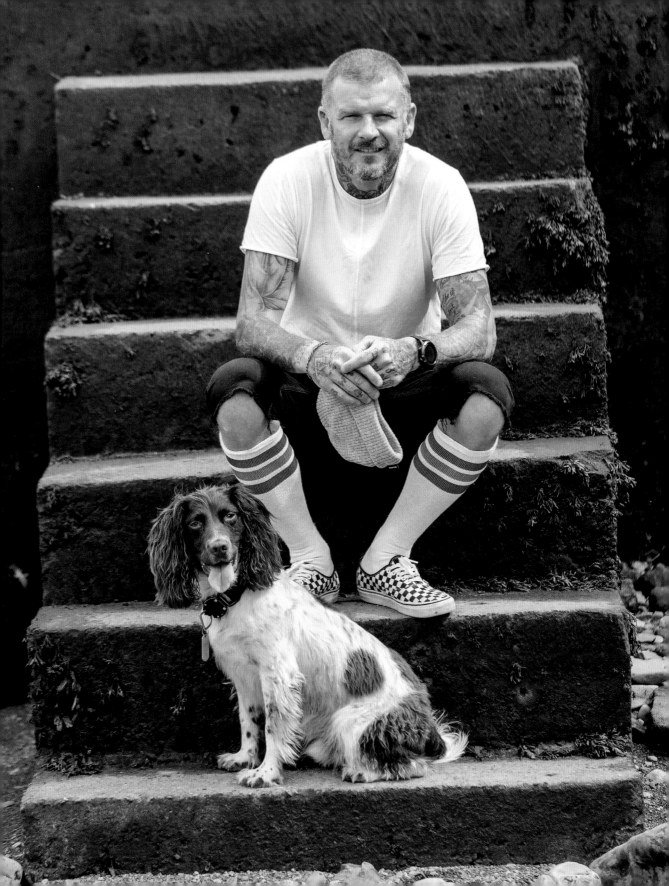

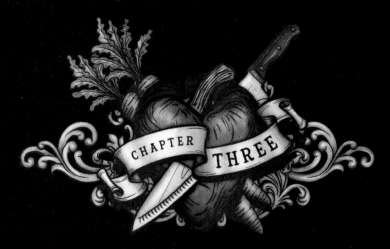

CHAPTER THREE

HOME COMFORT CLASSICS

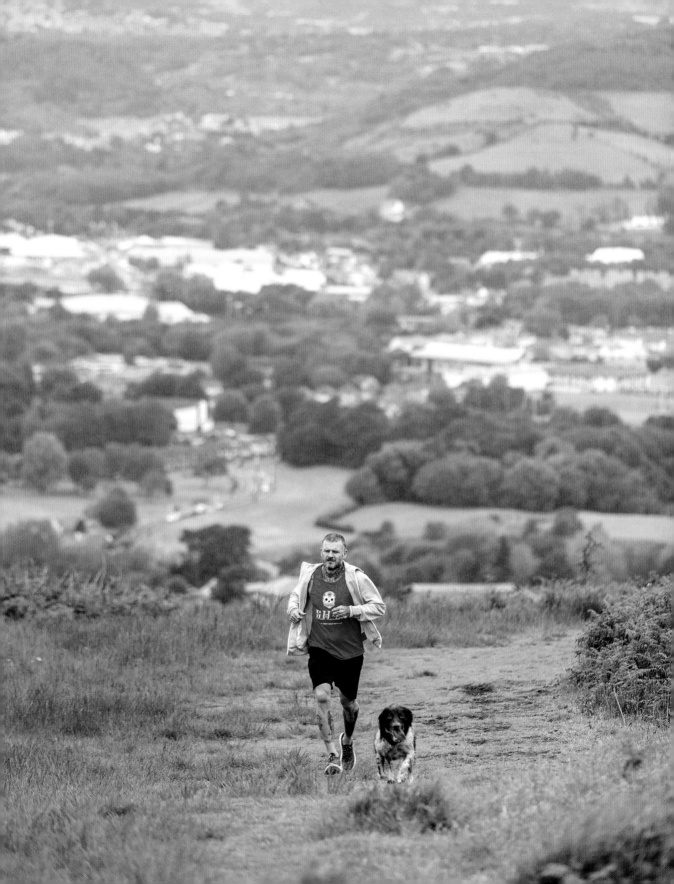

My main monthly outgoings are on food, both to eat and to experiment with. Like I've said, my mother always taught us to eat healthy food, so I was brought up with that engraved on my mind. We would, of course, also have comfort food days – which in our case consisted of the famous sausage, beans and chips – but a little bit of that here and there is all good when you do it in the right balance. Every kid loves comfort food days and me and my brothers were no different to anyone else. Back then, we had £1 pocket money, but we weren't allowed to spend it on sweets or chocolate. As you get older though, you take charge of your own eating habits, as your mam isn't there to inspect what you've bought with your money! If I'm honest, I went all out on sweet stuff and chocolates, as I'd been starved of them for so many years. I had a really sweet tooth up until my late 20s, and I think that's why I enjoyed creating puddings (and excelled at it) when I was at catering college.

As I got older, my taste buds changed and now I'm more of a savoury person, but I still love my comfort food. As an ultra-endurance athlete who trains quite a bit, I'm pretty lucky that I can eat all these calories and then just burn them away. I'm far from 'ripped', but I don't go for that look, as I need a little fat around the edges to burn in order to fuel my long-distance swims, bike rides or runs. Which is just as well! Casseroles, stews, sandwiches, chillies and curries are among my fave comfort food dishes and I love cooking them. Washing them down with one, two, maybe three glasses – ahhhhhhh, screw it, a whole bottle – of wine is another comfort. Cooking while drinking wine is one of life's great pleasures, they just go together so well that – before you know it – a bottle has gone... oops. And we all know that there is no comfort food like hangover comfort food either, they are very good friends, but again, all in moderation.

Today I try my best to eat a wholesome fruit and veg-based diet, cutting out the processed foods (even with a hangover), but I'd be lying if I said I did it all the time. After all, I'm human like the rest of you and if life's little processed or comfort food luxuries put that smile on your face when you need it, then jump in head-first. Just try not to jump in head-first every day...

VEGAN IRISH STEW TO GET DOWN YOU

SERVES 4–6

1 tablespoon olive oil
1 onion, finely chopped
2 garlic cloves, finely chopped
4 celery sticks, finely chopped
300g mushrooms, sliced
1 tablespoon tomato purée
3 medium potatoes,
    finely chopped
2 parsnips, finely chopped
2 carrots, finely chopped
½ swede, finely chopped
440ml can of Guinness,
    or other Irish stout
500ml vegetable stock
    (for homemade, see page 121)
1 tablespoon dried rosemary
1 tablespoon dried thyme
1 tablespoon cornflour
salt and pepper

I look at Dublin as my second home, as my fiancée of nine years lives there and I've been back and forth for all that time. I love Ireland, the people and their food-and-pub culture. One of my fave places to go is Johnnie Fox's pub, which must be one of Ireland's highest pubs, as it is way up in the Dublin mountains. It can be a bit touristy, but if you visit during the day it's very peaceful; I usually sit and have a Guinness with my dog Lemmy, but I enjoy this stew with a tot of Irish whiskey instead, as there's already nearly a pint of the black stuff in it!

Heat the oil in a large saucepan over a medium heat, add the onion and garlic and cook until soft but not coloured. Add the celery, mushrooms and tomato purée and cook until they, too, are soft, then add all the remaining vegetables and mix.

Pour in the Guinness and stock along with the rosemary and thyme and leave to simmer for 1 hour, until all the veg are tender.

Mix the cornflour in a small bowl with a little water to make a loose paste and add to the mixture, then simmer for a while to allow the stew to thicken. Season with salt and pepper to taste. You won't need anything on the side with this: everything you need is there!

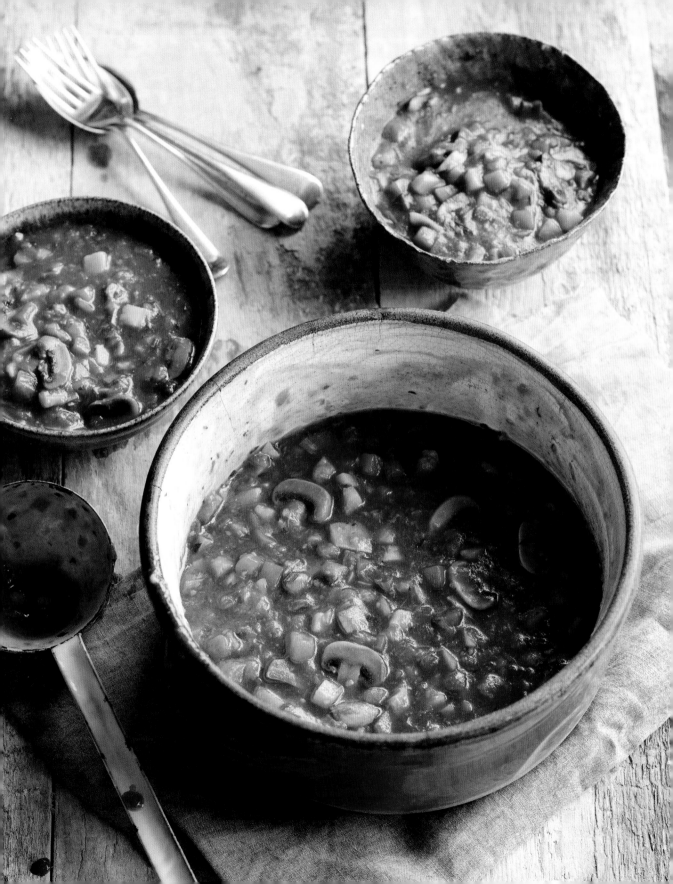

CREAMY MUSHROOM PRITCHANOFF

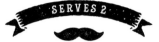

SERVES 2

1 tablespoon vegetable oil
2 onions, finely chopped
4 garlic cloves, finely chopped
500g mushrooms
　　(an assortment, if you wish)
3 tablespoons plain flour
1.2 litres vegetable stock
　　(for homemade, see page 121)
a few thyme sprigs
leaves from a bunch
　　of parsley, chopped
1 tablespoon vegan
　　Worcestershire sauce
　　(no worries if you haven't
　　got any, just leave it out)
1 tablespoon cider vinegar
200ml soya or oat cream
rice, to serve

Mushrooms, mushrooms, mushrooms, I could eat them until I turned into one. I love them raw or cooked and chestnut mushrooms are my favourite. If you love the good ol' mushroom too, then this dish is for you, as it's packed full of the buggers.

Heat the oil in a frying pan over a medium-low heat, add the onions and garlic and cook until softened but not browned.

Add the mushrooms and cook for a further 5 minutes, then add the flour. Cook the flour out for a few minutes – you may find it sticks to the pan a bit, but don't worry as next up is the veg stock. As soon as you add the veg stock, keep stirring to scrape the bits from the bottom of the pan and you'll find the sauce is thickening.

Add the thyme sprigs (you can remove them later) most of the parsley, the vegan Worcestershire sauce (if you have any), cider vinegar and soya or oat cream, bring to the boil, then reduce the heat and leave to simmer for 15 minutes. Remove the thyme sprigs, if you want.

Serve with rice.

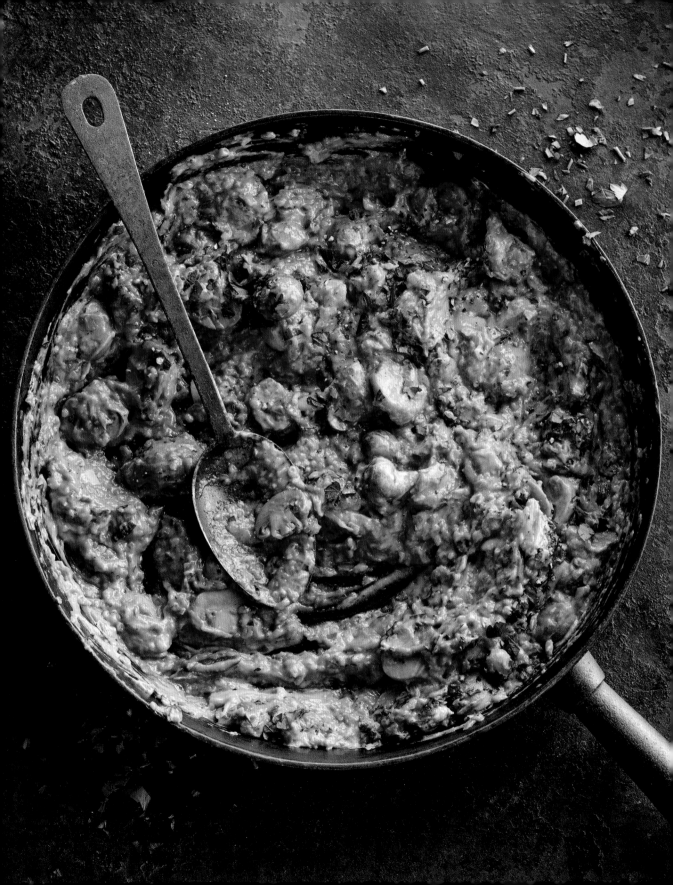

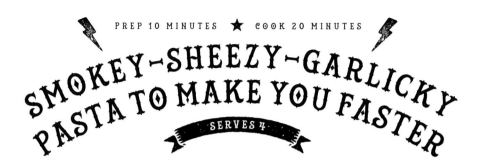

SMOKEY-SHEEZY-GARLICKY PASTA TO MAKE YOU FASTER

SERVES 4

150g broccoli, broken
   into florets
150g French beans
handful of frozen peas
500g pasta
400g cashew nuts,
   soaked overnight
100g silken tofu
2 teaspoons liquid smoke
1 garlic clove
5 tablespoons nutritional yeast
1 tablespoon smoked paprika
1 teaspoon celery salt
pepper
400ml unsweetened oat milk

*Carb up, carb up, because the last ride's the fast ride!
If you want to swim/bike/run fast, then you'd better have
the carbs to fuel that machine of yours called the human
body, which this recipe provides, plus the tofu gives you
the protein you need to repair your muscles. It not only
tastes banging, it's the perfect fuel for training or racing,
so get it down you the night before you need it.*

Bring a saucepan of water to the boil. Tip in the broccoli
florets and French beans and cook for 2–3 minutes, dropping
in the peas for the final 30 seconds (you want the peas
to just defrost and warm through, so they are still bright
green and sweet). Drain all the green veg.

Cook the pasta in boiling water according to the packet
instructions (different pastas take differing lengths
of time to cook through). Drain.

Meanwhile, get a food processor or (ideally) a powerful
blender and add the drained cashews, tofu, liquid smoke,
garlic, nutritional yeast, smoked paprika and celery salt,
then season generously with black pepper. Pulse a few
times until broken down. Slowly add the oat milk and
keep blending until you get a creamy texture.

Mix the smokey cream, pasta and green veg together
in a saucepan over a medium heat until piping hot all
the way through. Wait for it to go down, then jump
on yer bike and pedal up a steep hill…

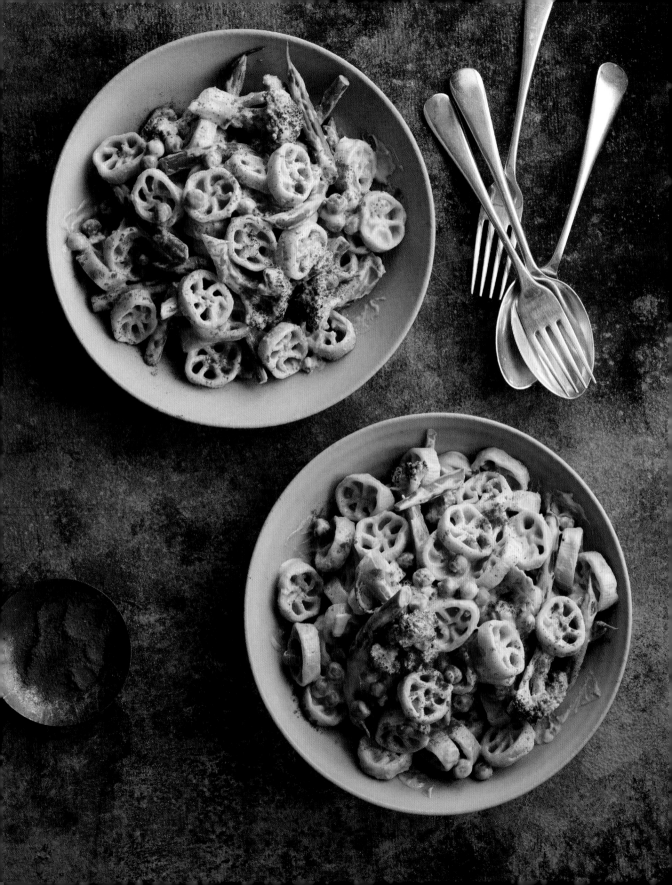

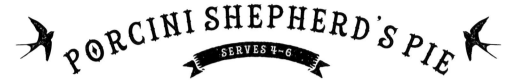

PORCINI SHEPHERD'S PIE

SERVES 4–6

20g dried porcini mushrooms
400ml warm water
4 tablespoons olive oil
2 carrots, finely chopped
2 celery sticks, finely chopped
1 onion, finely chopped
2 garlic cloves, finely chopped
2 bay leaves
200g green lentils
400g can chopped tomatoes
2 tablespoons soy sauce
1 tablespoon balsamic vinegar
700g floury potatoes, such as
    King Edward or Maris Piper,
    roughly chopped
1 tablespoon wholegrain mustard
50g dairy-free spread
salt and pepper

This has got to be the ultimate comfort food. Apart from a few easy-to-find fresh ingredients, most of it can be rustled together from your kitchen cupboard without fuss or fancy techniques. The dried porcini give a rich, umami flavour, but if you have other dried wild mushrooms, use those instead.

Cover the dried porcini with the measured warm water and set aside for 30 minutes.

Heat the olive oil in a large saucepan and, when it starts to shimmer, add the chopped carrots, celery and onion, along with a large pinch of salt. Cook over a low heat, uncovered, stirring occasionally, for 25 minutes, until everything is soft and the onion and celery are translucent.

Add the garlic and bay leaves and cook for a minute more. Drain the mushrooms through a sieve over a bowl, roughly chop and add them to the saucepan with their soaking liquid. Stir in the lentils and tomatoes. Fill the tomato can twice with water and add to the pan with the soy sauce and balsamic vinegar. Bring to the boil, then reduce the heat to a simmer. Cook for 30 minutes, until the lentils are soft and most of liquid has been absorbed. Season to taste.

Meanwhile, place the potatoes in a pan and cover with cold water. Bring to the boil and cook for 15–20 minutes, until a knife passes through the potatoes easily. Drain and mash with the mustard and spread until smooth. Season well.

Preheat the oven to 200°C (Gas Mark 6). Tip the lentil mixture into a 20 x 20cm baking tin, then spread the mashed potatoes over the top. Cook in the hot oven for 35–40 minutes, until golden on top and bubbling at the sides.

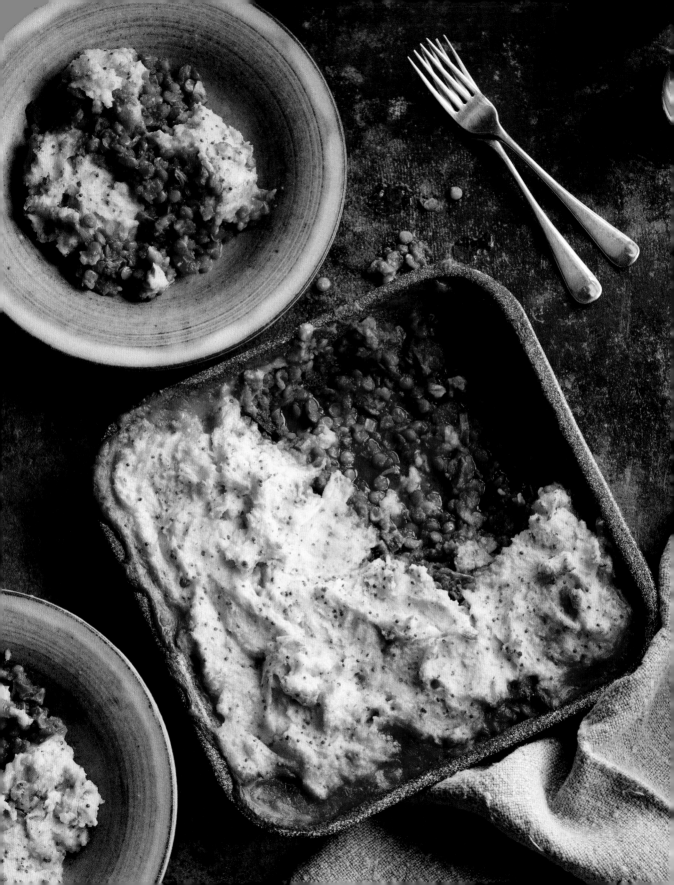

BRINED & BARBECUED RAINBOW ROOT VEG

SERVES 4 AS A SIDE

For the brine
750ml water
250ml cider vinegar
2 cloves
2 bay leaves
4 black peppercorns
10 coriander seeds
zest of ½ orange, pared
   off with a veg peeler
40g sugar
1 tablespoon sea salt

For the vegetables
300g mixed beetroots,
   unpeeled but well-scrubbed
300g mixed carrots, peeled and
   cut into irregular 3cm pieces
150g celeriac, peeled and roughly
   sliced into 3cm pieces
150g radishes, halved

For the herb oil
50ml extra virgin olive oil
leaves from a small bunch
   of basil

Brining vegetables before cooking them is a really surprising way to serve them. The brine not only softens root vegetables but also gives them a bright flavour packed with all the character of the aromatic spices and citrus peel it contains. Try these as part of a summer barbecue feast (see page 184), or stuffed into pitta breads with tahini and falafel.

Put all the brine ingredients in a large saucepan along with the beetroots. Bring to the boil, then reduce the heat to a simmer and cook for 10 minutes. Lift out the beetroots and run them under cold water. Rub the skins off and set aside.

Next, add the carrots and celeriac to the pan and cook gently for 5 minutes. Remove with a slotted spoon and pat dry with kitchen paper. The celeriac and carrots will be stained slightly pink from the beetroot, but this looks great on the plate. Finally, lower the radishes into the brine and cook for 3 minutes. Remove from the pan and pat dry.

Barbecue all the brined vegetables over a medium heat for 3–5 minutes each side, until smoky and charred in places. If you don't have a barbecue, heat a griddle pan over a high heat for at least 5 minutes before charring the vegetables in batches for 5 minutes on each side. Either way, take care not to move them around too much – this helps the char marks to form and the smoky flavour to develop. When the vegetables are cooked, transfer them to a warm platter.

Whizz the oil and basil in a blender or food processor and drizzle it over the vegetables.

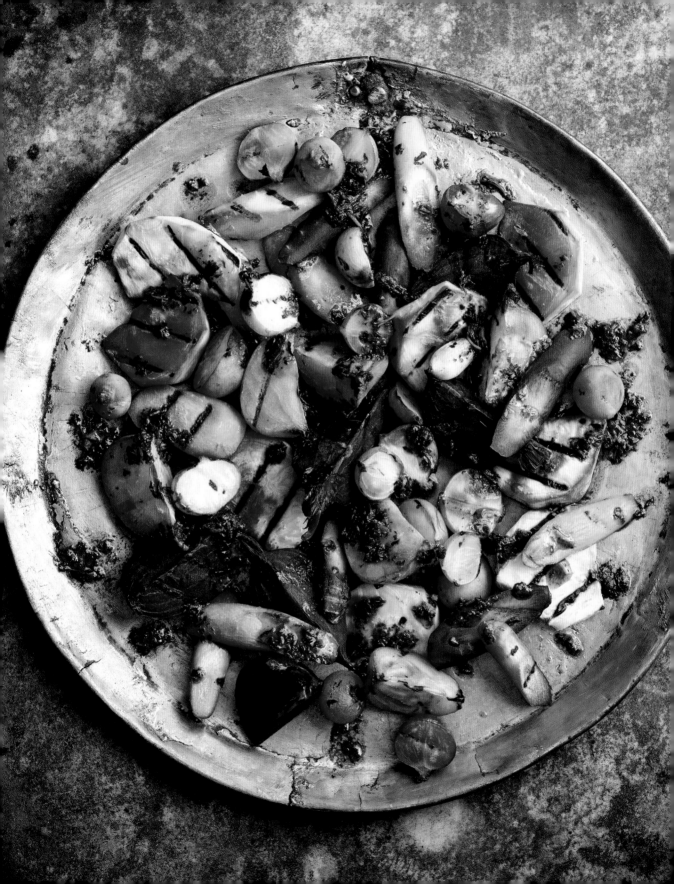

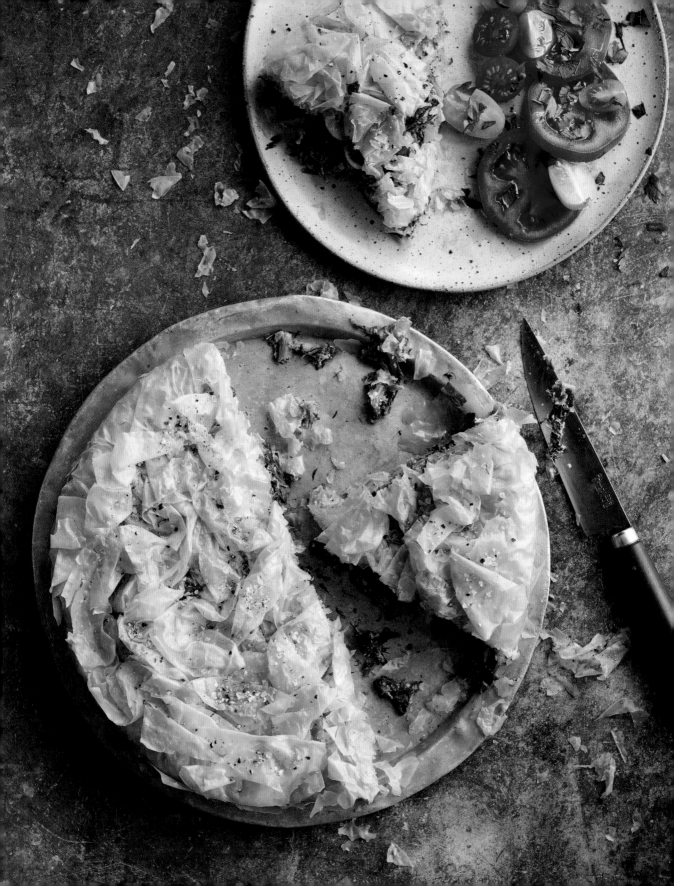

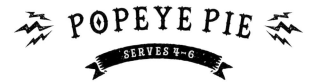

POPEYE PIE

SERVES 4–6

50g cashew nuts
750g greens (I like a mix
    of spinach, kale, chard
    and spring greens)
2 tablespoons flavourless oil,
    such as mild olive oil
small bunch of spring onions,
    thinly sliced
4 garlic cloves, thinly sliced
300g silken tofu
1 nutmeg
½ teaspoon sea salt flakes
leaves from a bunch of parsley,
    roughly chopped
leaves from a bunch of dill,
    roughly chopped
100g pitted green olives,
    roughly chopped
salt and pepper
100g dairy-free spread, melted
8 filo pastry sheets

*Packed with leafy green vegetables, this pie is bursting
with iron and brimming with amazing mineral flavour.
Popeye would be lost without Olive, so, of course, there
are salty pops of green olive throughout the filling too.*

Place the cashew nuts in a bowl and cover with hot water.
Leave to soak for at least 30 minutes.

Wash the greens in plenty of cold water, then, while the leaves
are still wet, put them in a large saucepan and cover with
a lid. Place over a medium heat until they wilt (this should
take about 5 minutes). Transfer the greens to a colander
over the kitchen sink and allow the leaves to cool and
the steam to evaporate.

Meanwhile, heat the oil in a small frying pan over a medium
heat. Tip the spring onions and garlic into the pan and cook
for 5 minutes, until completely soft and just beginning to
colour. Transfer to a large mixing bowl.

Squeeze as much water from the greens as you can. Roughly
chop and add to the bowl with the spring onions and garlic.

Preheat the oven to 180°C (Gas Mark 4).

Drain the cashew nuts and place in a food processor with
the tofu. Grate in one-eighth of the nutmeg and add the sea
salt flakes. Process until the mixture has the consistency of
thick yogurt. Stir the tofu mixture into the bowl of greens,
along with the herbs and olives and season generously.

Recipe continues overleaf

Brush a 23cm springform tin all over with the melted dairy-free spread. Lay a sheet of filo over the tin (keeping the remaining sheets covered under a tea towel to prevent them cracking and drying out). Brush the filo in the tin with melted spread, leaving the sheet overhanging, before giving the tin a quarter turn and laying over another filo sheet, brushing again with melted spread. Repeat with 4 more sheets, saving 2 for the top. Pack the greens into the base and smooth over with a spatula. Unfold the overhanging filo corners over the filling, brushing each edge with melted spread as you go. Arrange the remaining 2 filo sheets on top in ruffled bunches and brush again with spread.

Bake for 45 minutes until deep golden all over. Allow to cool in the tin for 15 minutes before removing it. The filling will still be hot, but this will help the mixture to set, making it much easier to slice.

GUEST CHEF: LENTIL SLOPPY JOES

SERVES 6

For the Sloppy Joes

1 tablespoon olive oil
2 garlic cloves, crushed
½ white onion, finely chopped
½ red pepper, finely chopped
½ teaspoon cayenne pepper (optional)
400g cooked lentils (we use Puy)
250g tomato sauce
2 tablespoons soy sauce
2 tablespoons tomato purée
1 tablespoon brown sugar
1 teaspoon paprika
1 tablespoon balsamic vinegar

For the wedges

3 large sweet potatoes, well scrubbed, cut into wedges
2 tablespoons olive oil
2 teaspoons smoked paprika
1 garlic clove, crushed
salt and pepper

To serve (everything except the buns are optional!)

hamburger buns
pickled gherkins
carrot ribbons
pickled red cabbage
chilli slices
avocado slices

Sloppy Joes don't make much sense on paper – it's basically a sort of spag bol sauce in a roll! It totally works though. This plant-based recipe comes from Laura Graham of Tidy Kitchen in Cardiff who has kept me fed through many a TV shoot! What would I do without her?!

Preheat the oven to 200°C (Gas Mark 6). Heat the oil for the Sloppy Joes in a frying pan over a medium heat. Add all the chopped vegetables and the cayenne pepper, if using, and fry, pouring in 2 tablespoons of water to prevent catching. Cook slowly to ensure the vegetables soften and don't burn; it should take about 15 minutes.

Add all the remaining ingredients and stir. Cook over a medium-low heat for about 20 minutes, or until the sauce thickens. This is all about a long slow cook; love the sloppy joe and it will love you.

Meanwhile, put the sweet potato wedges in a roasting tin with the oil, paprika, garlic and salt and pepper. Put the wedges in the oven and cook for about 30 minutes, turning halfway through, or until tender.

When the sauce and wedges are nearly ready, toast the hamburger buns. Taste the sauce and adjust the seasoning with salt and pepper. Serve the Sloppy Joe filling over the toasted buns and top with your choice of pickled gherkins, carrot ribbons, pickled red cabbage, freshly sliced chillies and avocado. Don't forget the sweet potato wedges.

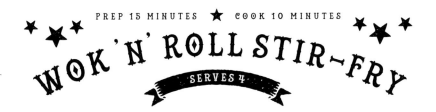

WOK 'N' ROLL STIR-FRY

SERVES 4

1 tablespoon sunflower oil
4 garlic cloves, sliced
60g fresh root ginger,
    cut into thin batons
2 red onions, sliced
2 red peppers, sliced
200g mangetout
100g baby sweetcorn
100g courgettes, sliced
2 spring onions, sliced
handful of peanuts
noodles, to serve (optional)

For the sauce
3 tablespoons soy sauce
1 tablespoon rice vinegar
1 tablespoon maple syrup
    or agave syrup
1½ tablespoons cornflour

We all love a good stir-fry. This version has a thicker sauce for that Chinese takeaway feel and peanuts for a hit of crunch. Get in from work after a busy day, crack open a bottle of beer or wine, chill out, then hit the kitchen, knife in hand, veg ready to be chopped and wok on a high heat. Literally in 10 minutes you've got a super-healthy meal to eat. You can wash it all down with that super-healthy beer or wine too. Ahem.

Make sure you have everything prepped and ready, as this should be fast, hot cooking, otherwise the veg will just get soggy, not crisp. Mix all the ingredients for the sauce in a small bowl.

Heat up the wok over a high heat and add the oil. When the oil is hot, add the garlic and ginger, keeping it constantly moving to stop it from burning. Add the red onions and soften, then add the peppers, mangetout, baby sweetcorn, courgettes and spring onions and constantly mix all the ingredients in the wok to stop anything from burning. If you've seen a Chinese chef cook in a restaurant before, you'll notice he/she's constantly working the wok.

Do not overcook the veg, as you really want it to be crunchy. Add the sauce you mixed earlier to the wok and stir into the veg until thickened. Sprinkle with the peanuts and eat on its own, or add to noodles.

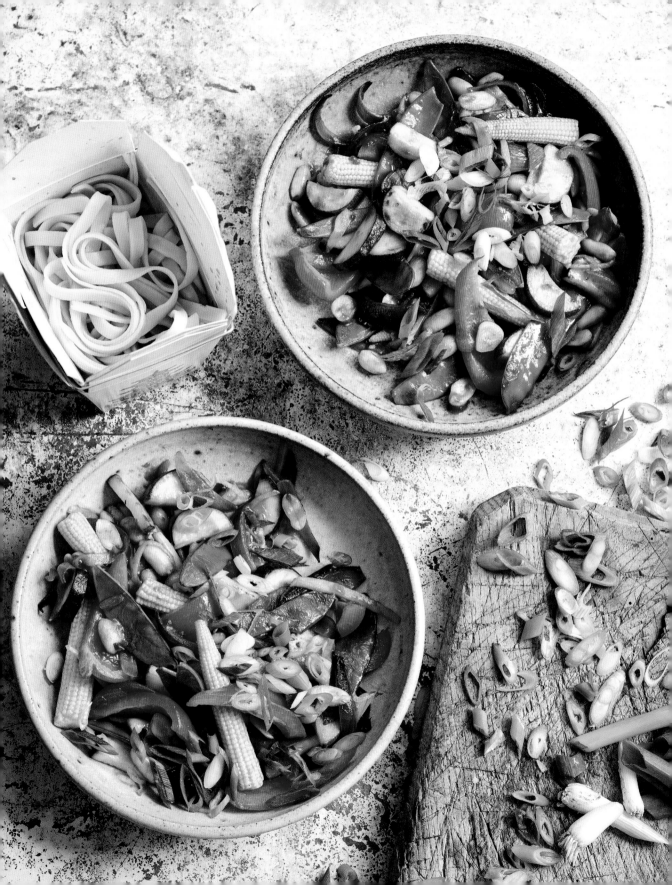

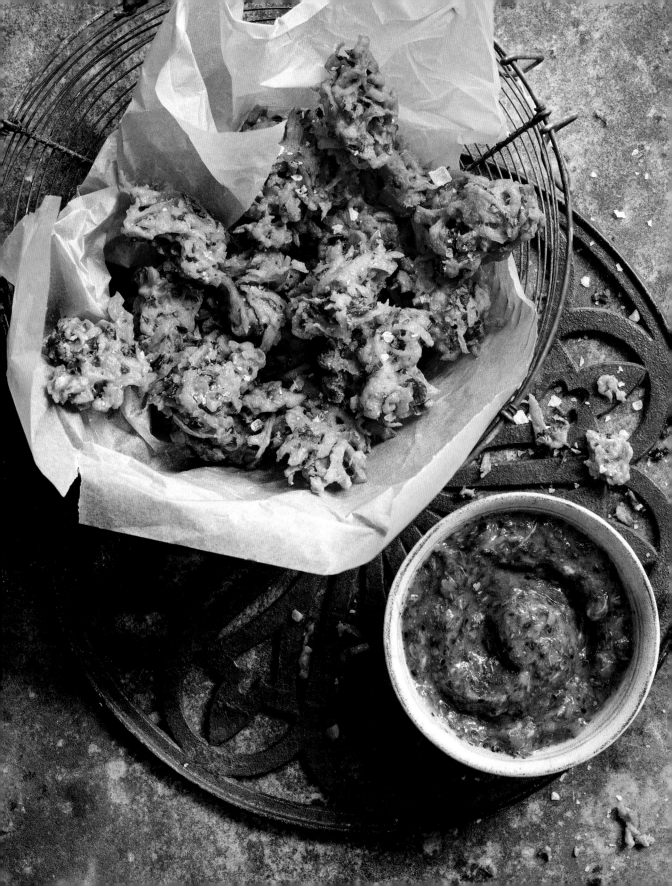

CARROT & HERB PAKORAS WITH MANGO & HERB CHUTNEY

SERVES 4

For the chutney

1 teaspoon cumin seeds
½ teaspoon black mustard seeds
½ mango, peeled and roughly
    chopped (about 150g
    prepared weight)
1 green chilli, deseeded
    and roughly chopped
2 garlic cloves, roughly chopped
2 tablespoons rice wine vinegar
1 teaspoon salt
juice of 1 lime
10g fresh root ginger,
    peeled and finely grated
leaves from ½ bunch of coriander
leaves from ½ bunch of mint

For the pakoras

flavourless vegetable oil,
    for deep-frying
3 carrots, grated
1 small onion, grated
1 teaspoon garam masala
½ teaspoon asafoetida
    (optional, see recipe
    introduction)
leaves from ½ bunch of coriander
leaves from ½ bunch of mint
75g gram (chickpea) flour
sea salt flakes

Don't be put off trying to cook these by the exotic name; pakora is essentially an Indian term for 'fritter'. These crispy little pakoras use gram flour (made from chickpeas), making the mix gluten-free as well as protein-rich. Asafoetida is optional, but is available from most large supermarkets and Asian supermarkets. While the name sounds like someone has sneezed, it imparts a deeply savoury flavour and is a great digestive aid, as it combats the (ahem) negative effects of lots of fibre from pulses and leafy vegetables.

First, make the chutney. Toast the cumin seeds and mustard seeds in a dry frying pan until incredibly fragrant and the mustard seeds start to pop. Tip into a saucepan with all the other chutney ingredients except the herbs, cover and cook over a medium heat for 15 minutes, adding a splash of water if the mango looks as though it's catching on the pan. Allow to cool for 5 minutes, then scrape everything from the pan into a food processor. Add the coriander and mint and whizz into a bright green chutney. Transfer to a bowl and set aside.

Heat an 8cm depth of vegetable oil in a saucepan over a medium heat (make sure the oil comes no more than one-third of the way up the pan, for safety reasons).

Recipe continues overleaf

Meanwhile, toss the grated carrot and onion with the spices, then add the herbs and mix to combine. Sift the gram flour into the bowl, then add up to 150ml water, a little at a time, mixing as you go, to create a thick batter that coats all the vegetables.

Test to see if the oil is hot enough; if a drop of batter bubbles vigorously and rises to the surface immediately, the oil is ready. Drop spoonfuls of the pakora mixture into the hot oil, frying no more than 4 at a time, and use a slotted spoon to turn them after 2 minutes of cooking. Cook for a further minute on the other side, then lift the pakoras out with a slotted spoon and drain on kitchen paper. Repeat to cook all the pakoras.

While the pakoras are cooling, sprinkle over sea salt flakes. If you want to keep them warm for a while before serving without them going soggy, keep them in a low oven with the door left slightly ajar.

Serve the pakoras with the chutney on the side.

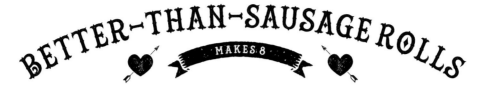

BETTER-THAN-SAUSAGE ROLLS

MAKES 8

20g dried mushrooms

50g pearled barley, cooked according to the packet instructions

50g dairy-free spread, plus extra for brushing and greasing

4 shallots, finely chopped

3 garlic cloves, crushed

200g Portobello mushrooms, finely chopped

100ml dry sherry or white wine

leaves from 5 thyme sprigs

1 teaspoon ground mace

1 teaspoon fennel seeds, plus extra for sprinkling

1 teaspoon chia seeds

50g Cheddar-style vegan cheese, grated

500g block of vegan puff pastry

plain flour, for dusting

salt and pepper

Ahh... sausage rolls! These really are better than the original – like a hug in your mouth. Don't be tempted to scrimp on the wine or spices here; the filling mixture is given a complex depth by each ingredient. Chia seeds are used to bind the filling in the same way as egg, but ground flax seeds would work too. Most shop-bought puff pastries are vegan, unless they state 'all butter' on the packaging, so do check on the packet to be sure. If you want to make these ahead of time, freeze them, then bake from frozen for 35–40 minutes, covering with foil if they look as though they may burn.

Cover the dried mushrooms with warm water and set aside for 30 minutes. Place the cooked pearl barley in a large mixing bowl.

Melt half the dairy-free spread in a large frying pan (I use a 28cm one) and fry the shallots with a pinch of salt over a low heat for 5–7 minutes, until soft and translucent. Add the garlic and cook for a further 2 minutes. Scrape the shallot mixture into the mixing bowl with the barley and wipe out the pan with a piece of kitchen paper.

Return to the pan to the heat and melt the remaining spread. Cook the chopped mushrooms with a pinch of salt, stirring regularly until all the liquid from the mushrooms has evaporated and they are golden all over. Drain and roughly chop the dried mushrooms and add these, along with the sherry or wine, and simmer until all the liquid has been absorbed. Stir in the thyme, mace and fennel and season well with salt and pepper. Stir through the chia seeds while the mixture is still warm.

Recipe continues overleaf

Tip the mushroom mixture into the bowl with the barley and add the cheese. Taste and adjust the seasoning, adding a touch more black pepper than you think you need.

Slice the puff pastry block in half and, on a lightly floured surface, roll the pastry into 2 rough 30 x 15cm rectangles. Brush each pastry rectangle with melted spread.

Arrange half the mushroom mixture 2cm from the edge of a pastry rectangle, forming a 4cm mound of filling down the length of the pastry and leaving about 9cm of pastry on the other side. Fold the pastry from the 9cm edge over the mushrooms and press down to seal (with the prongs of a fork to make an attractive pattern, if you wish). Brush with melted spread and sprinkle with fennel seeds and more black pepper. Repeat with the remaining pastry and mushroom mixture.

Slide each pie on to a baking sheet lined with baking parchment and chill for at least 30 minutes. (Or freeze them at this point, *see* recipe introduction).

Preheat the oven to 220°C (Gas Mark 7).

Remove the rolls from the fridge and cut each into 4 sausage roll shapes. Place on a lightly greased baking sheet. Bake for 20–25 minutes, until deep golden all over.

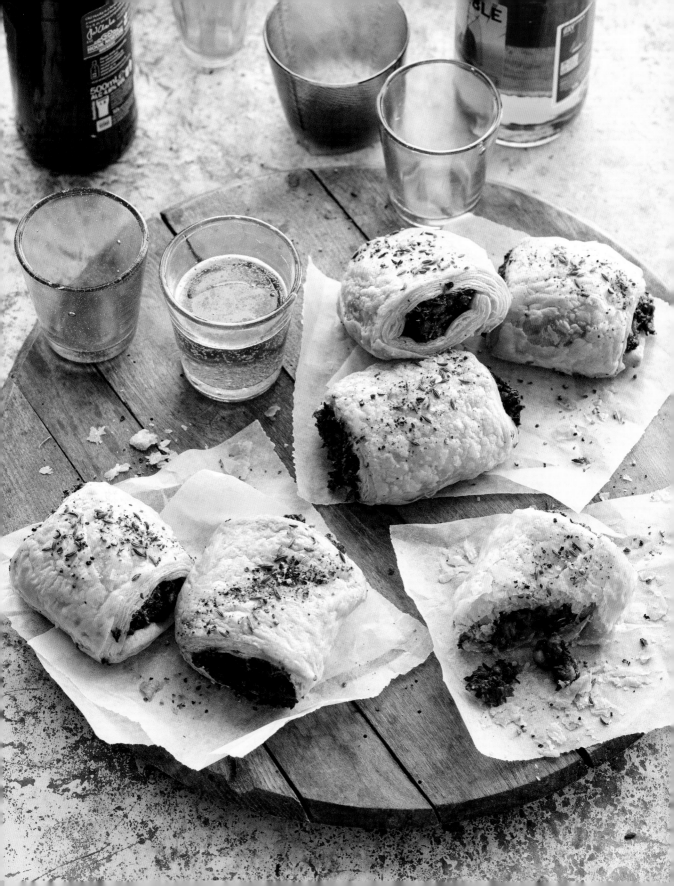

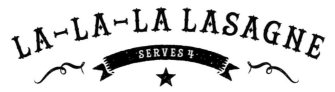

LA-LA-LA LASAGNE

SERVES 4

To assemble
6–9 egg-free lasagne sheets,
    depending how many
    layers you want
splash of olive oil
200g pack vegan mozzarella,
    or other vegan cheese, grated

For the creamy sauce
300g cashew nuts, soaked
    overnight in water
6 tablespoons nutritional yeast
1 teaspoon miso
1 teaspoon garlic salt
1 teaspoon smoked paprika
240ml unsweetened oat milk

For the tomato sauce
2 tablespoons olive oil
2 onions, finely chopped
3 garlic cloves, finely chopped
3 celery sticks, finely chopped
1 red pepper, finely chopped
200g mushrooms, finely
    chopped or sliced
650g tomato passata
400g can borlotti, cannellini
    or black-eyed beans, drained
1 tablespoon dried oregano
1 vegetable stock cube
1 tablespoon balsamic vinegar
1 teaspoon maple syrup
100g baby spinach

*When eating a mouthful of this, close your eyes and
pretend you're on a gondola in Venice, but let the lasagne
sing to you instead of a gondolier. The creamy sauce here
will work best if you have a powerful blender to really
bash the living daylights out of the cashew nuts.*

Cook the lasagne in boiling water, adding the splash
of oil, then drain and lay out on a plate, then set aside.

Drain the cashews and put them in a powerful blender.
Add the nutritional yeast, miso, garlic salt and smoked
paprika and blitz for a few seconds, then slowly start
adding the oat milk, until you get a creamy sauce.

To make the tomato sauce, heat the oil in a frying pan over
a medium heat. Fry the onions, garlic and celery until soft
but not coloured, then add the red pepper and mushrooms
and cook through, stirring the mixture every so often, for
about 5 minutes. Add the passata, beans, oregano and stock
cube and mix, then pour in the balsamic and maple syrup.
Let the sauce simmer for a good 30 minutes. Finally, stir
in the spinach leaves and allow them to wilt.

Time to start putting it all together. Preheat the oven to
180°C (Gas Mark 4). Put a decent amount of the tomato
sauce on the bottom of an ovenproof dish. Now layer on
a little bit of the cashew sauce, then cover with lasagne
sheets. Repeat this layering, making sure that the top
layer is just the tomato sauce and no cashew cream.

Sprinkle with the vegan mozzarella or other cheese
and bake for 45 minutes, or until bubbling and golden.

DIAL-IT-UP BROWN LENTIL DHAL

SERVES 4

300g brown lentils
2 tablespoons vegetable oil
2 tablespoons dairy-free spread
1 teaspoon mustard seeds
1 teaspoon cumin seeds
1 teaspoon ground coriander
1 teaspoon chilli powder
1 teaspoon ground turmeric
2 onions, finely chopped
5 garlic cloves, finely grated
1 chilli, or more, to taste
    (depending how hot you like
    your food), finely chopped
300ml vegetable stock
    (for homemade, see page 121)
250ml oat cream
salt and pepper
handful of coriander
    leaves, chopped
brown rice, to serve

Indian food rocks. Why? Because it's full of flavour and great spices that do wonders for the human body. As the saying goes, 'let food be thy medicine', and there's a lot of Indian recipes that have been known for centuries to be therapeutic. This recipe came about because I had a load of brown lentils in the cupboard that had been there for a while, so I decided to cook myself a dhal and I wasn't disappointed. It's proper comforting vegan Indian food.

Cook the brown lentils in some boiling water until soft, about 20 minutes, but check the packet instructions. Drain.

Meanwhile, heat the oil and dairy-free spread in a frying pan over a medium-high heat until it's really hot. Add the mustard seeds (they should be popping in the hot oil), cumin seeds, ground coriander, chilli powder and turmeric so you've got yourself a nice flavoured oil there. Add the onions and garlic to the pan; you should now be getting some great smells hovering around your kitchen.

Tip in the drained lentils, followed by the chilli and stock and cook for 15 minutes, letting those lentils soak up a bit of the stock. Add the oat cream and leave to simmer for a good hour, letting that sauce reduce a little while the lentils soak up those lovely flavours. Keep an eye on the sauce to make sure it isn't going too dry; the lentils should be left with a nice rich consistency.

Taste and adjust the seasoning, then scatter with coriander and serve with rice.

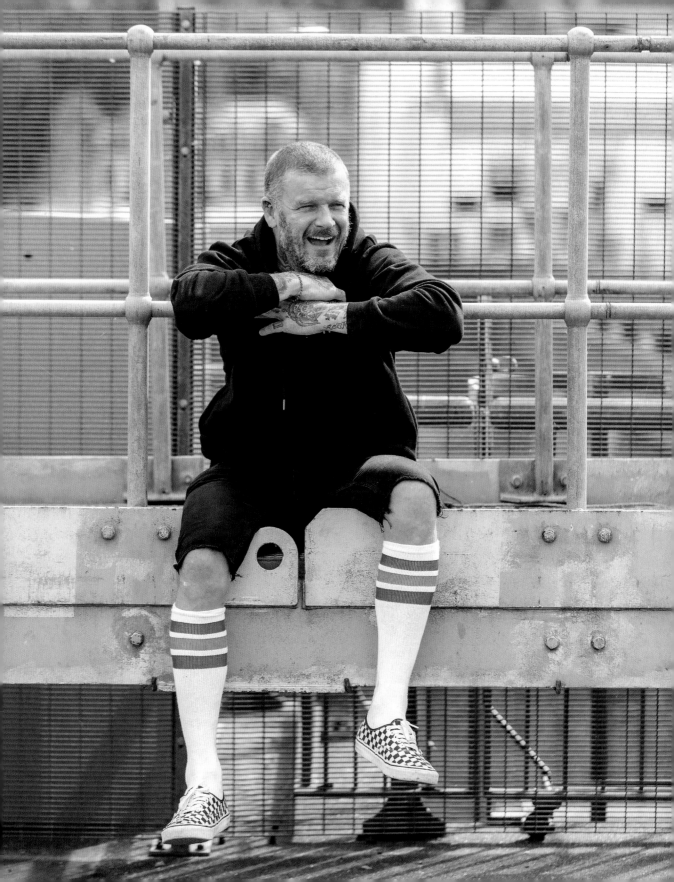

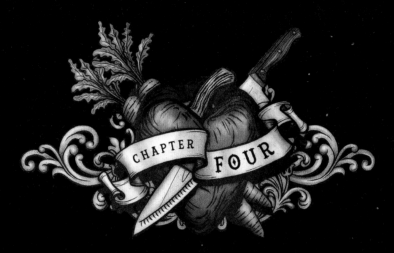

FOOD
WITH
LEGS

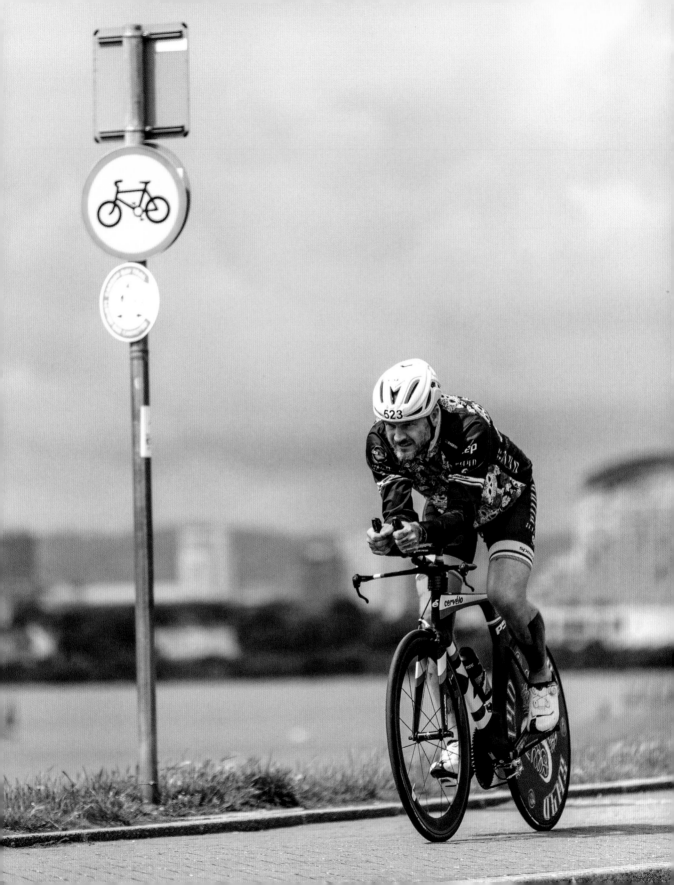

As I sit here writing this, I'm thinking back on the rock 'n' roll experiences I've amassed over the years, and I know I am lucky. I've been in some mental situations and my mind is full of them... or, I should say, hazily full of them, for obvious reasons. I've partied with the best of them and it's left me with a wealth of great stories. I'd love to share some of them with you, but I'm aware that a lot of the younger generation will be reading this, so I'll let you all use your imaginations!

There's a flip side, though, because it's also those experiences that pushed me to try another direction in life, due to the excess of it all. Narcotics, alcohol and lack of rest inevitably took my mind and body to a place I wasn't happy with... hence the dramatic turnaround in diet and lifestyle. Completing triathlons and honing my fitness were my new goals in life, not how many days I could stay awake, how much booze I could drink, or what volume of drugs I could take. Handily, the 'how long can I stay awake' challenge I used to put myself through is now proving itself useful when it comes to early training for endurance sports events, such as double and triple Ironman competitions!

But your body ain't gonna carry on unless you keep feeding it what it needs. A car will not move without petrol, oil and water and it's the same deal with your body... it screams for fuel. When I do my big fitness challenges, my fuel is dates, bananas, potatoes, pasta, nuts and raisins. The trick is to eat a hearty brekkie of porridge laced with bananas and maple syrup a good hour or so before starting exercise. However, that will not fire you up for the whole day, so it's a case of eating little but often... hence me munching on dates, which are full of carbs with a nice sweet kick. I'd also have smoothies, made from plant-based milks, fruit, hemp seeds and protein-packed tofu. The smoothies come in handy when you've been going strong for a good 10 hours or more: when you pass this point, trying to eat is very hard, as your body's so tired that you're just not in the mood for it at all. A smoothie goes down much more easily than solid food, giving you the vital nutrients you need to keep going.

At the end of the day, you can of course keep feeding fuel to that fire and your body will carry on moving... but what really keeps you going is your *mind*. If you have an unbalanced mind then, quite simply, you'll give up. I've learned the hard way that you may need to dig really deep to discover your determination and persistence, but you will find it; we can all surprise ourselves. It's not for everyone, but if you want to take on some physical challenges – or just fancy a run now and then – I've found that fitness is a far more positive way of keeping rocking than my past life's exploits.

The dishes in this chapter are designed with that in mind. They are filling but not soporific, to help you during your busy days. Let's face it, modern life can be a bit of a marathon in itself!

BÁHN MÌ (VIETNAMESE SARNIE) WITH TEMPEH and GREEN PÂTÉ

SERVES 2–EPICALLY

For the pickled veg
1 tablespoon palm sugar,
   or brown sugar
3 tablespoons rice vinegar
½ red onion, thinly sliced
1 carrot, cut into fine
   matchsticks
4 radishes, thinly sliced
¼ cucumber, cut into
   fine matchsticks
salt

For the pâté
150g frozen broad beans,
   defrosted
100g frozen peas, defrosted
1 garlic clove, chopped
stalks from a small bunch
   of coriander (use the
   leaves in the sarnie)
finely grated zest and juice
   of 1 lime

For the sarnie
1 tablespoon sriracha sauce
2 tablespoons vegan mayonnaise
2 tablespoons flavourless
   vegetable oil
200g marinated tempeh, sliced
   (Oasis brand is good)
2 small baguettes, or 1 large
   baguette, halved
leaves from the small bunch
   of coriander (from the pâté)
leaves from a small bunch of mint

This is an epic Scooby Doo sarnie and well worth the effort. Loads of Asian flavours, packed into a French baguette. Matchsticking the veg can be a pain, but you can buy julienne peelers for a few quid that do the job in a flash.

To pickle the veg, mix the sugar and vinegar together in a mixing bowl with a generous pinch of salt. Add the veg, mix it well and leave to pickle for at least 30 minutes, preferably overnight.

To make the pâté, put everything apart from the lime juice into a food processor or blender. Add half the lime juice and a pinch of salt, then blitz into a smooth paste. Taste and adjust the seasoning with more salt or lime juice or both, to your liking.

Mix the sriracha with the mayonnaise.

When the veg is ready, drain away any remaining vinegar.

Heat the oil in a frying pan over a medium-high heat. Fry the tempeh slices for 1–2 minutes a side, until nicely browned and cooked through.

Cut open your baguettes, or baguette halves. Slather the pâté on to one side and the hot mayo on to the other. Lay the tempeh in, followed by plenty of pickled veg. Finish by jamming in lots of freshly torn coriander and mint leaves.

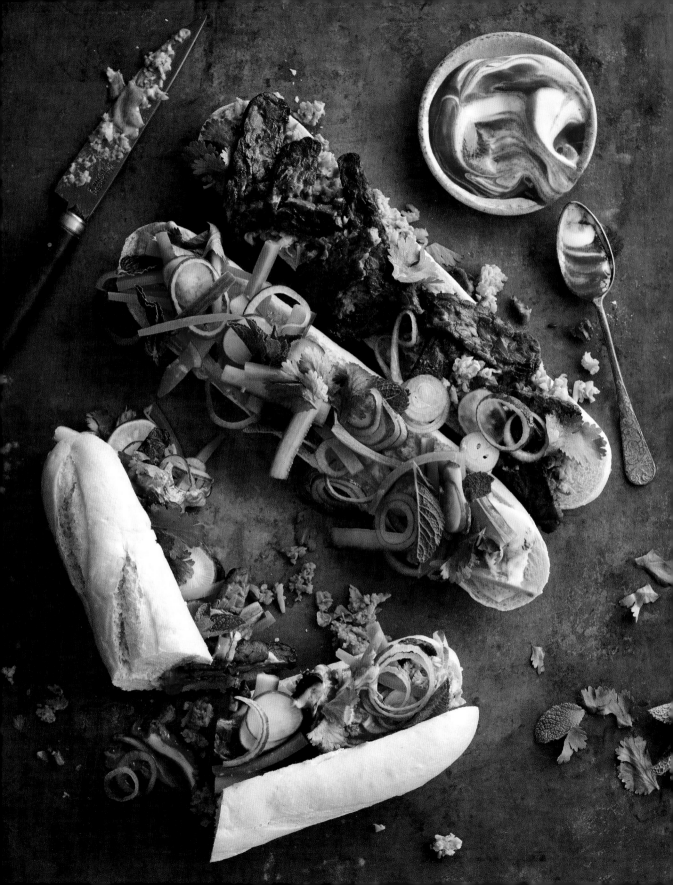

TEX MEX QUINOA SALAD WITH AVOCADO DRESSING

SERVES 2

120g quinoa
250g cherry tomatoes, halved
200g roasted red peppers, sliced
1 tablespoon chipotle paste,
    or to taste
1 tablespoon olive oil
2 spring onions, finely sliced
150g sweetcorn kernels
120g podded edamame beans,
    fresh or defrosted
small handful of mixed
    sprouted seeds
salt and pepper

For the dressing
1 avocado, peeled and pitted
½ garlic clove, finely chopped
small handful of coriander,
    coarse stalks removed
2 tablespoons lime juice
1 tablespoon olive oil

You can prep all the veg yourself from scratch if you like, but canned and jarred versions are easily available and speed things up no end. The veg is easily switchable, this is all about the dressing: creamy, herby and sweet. The avocados must be ripe, in fact this is an ideal use for any that feel a bit too soft for slicing.

Put a kettle on to boil. While you wait, rinse the quinoa in a sieve under cold running water.

Measure out 400ml boiling water into a saucepan. Tip in the quinoa and add a generous pinch of salt. Cook gently for 12–15 minutes, until tender.

While the quinoa cooks, mix the tomatoes and peppers together in a bowl with the chipotle paste, olive oil and a pinch of salt. Leave to macerate.

When the quinoa is ready, drain away any excess water and spread it out on a plate to cool down for 10 minutes.

To make the dressing, put everything into a food processor or blender and blitz until smooth. It will be very thick, so add some cold water, a little at a time, until it reaches a just-pourable yogurt-like consistency. Season well with salt.

Add the warm quinoa to the bowl with the tomatoes, followed by the spring onions, sweetcorn and edamame beans. Mix well and divide between 2 plates. Spoon the dressing artistically over the top and scatter with some sprouted seeds.

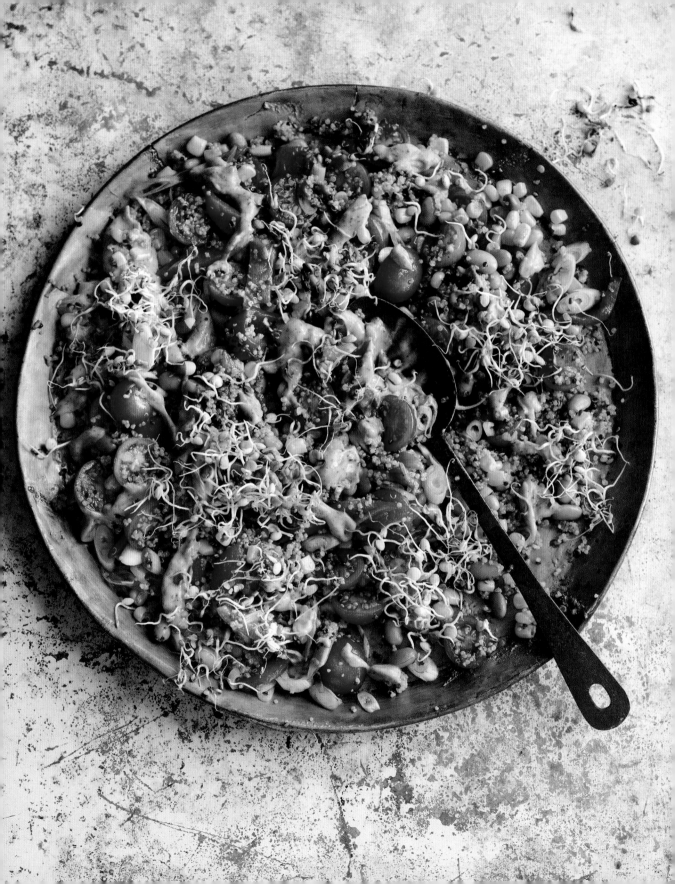

WHIPPED WHITE BEAN and ASPARAGUS TOASTS

SERVES 2

1 unwaxed lemon
400g can cannellini
  beans, drained
½ teaspoon ground cumin
½ garlic clove, finely chopped
2 tablespoons olive oil,
  plus extra for the asparagus
200g asparagus spears, trimmed
small bunch of parsley
30g toasted hazelnuts
2 slices of sourdough bread
salt and pepper

A comforting lunch, best made when the asparagus season is in full swing. If you have a griddle pan, then great. If not, you can always cook the asparagus spears in a frying pan, boil or steam them for a few minutes, or even roast them in a hot oven.

Put a griddle pan on to heat up. Finely zest half the lemon and set aside.

Tip the beans, cumin and garlic into a food processor or blender. Add the olive oil, a pinch of salt and a squeeze of lemon juice. Blitz into a smooth purée. Taste and tweak with a little more salt and lemon juice, to your liking.

Place your asparagus into the hot griddle pan and cook for 4–5 minutes, rolling occasionally, until tender and nicely marked. Remove from the pan, season them well and toss with a little oil to help the salt and pepper stick.

Pick the parsley leaves away from the stalks and chop them coarsely on a board with the hazelnuts, lemon zest and a small pinch of salt.

Toast the bread, in a toaster or in the griddle pan.

To serve, slather the toast with whipped beans and top with an unruly pile of asparagus. Garnish with plenty of the herb, zest and nut mixture.

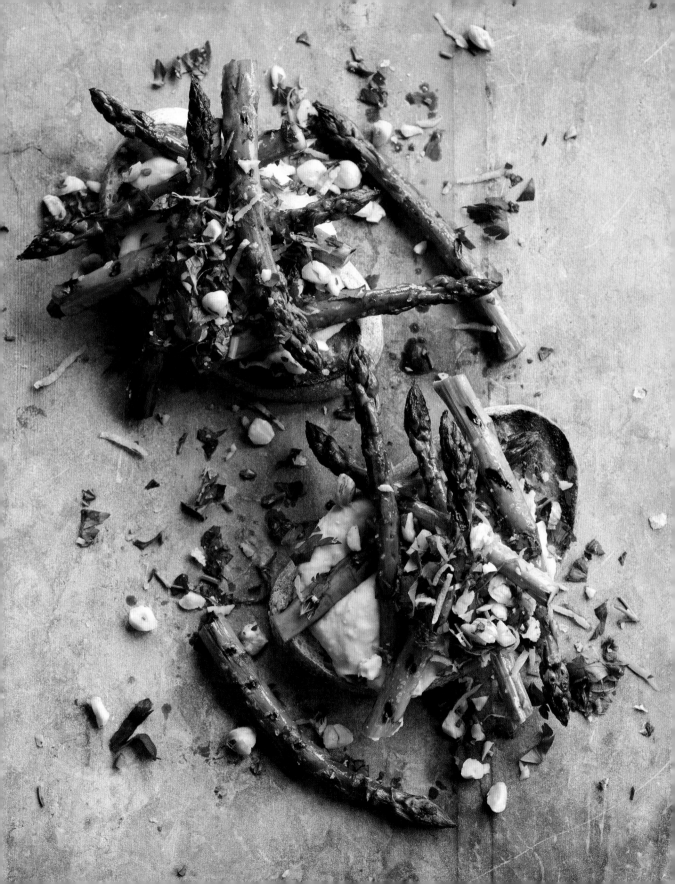

CAULIFLOWER FATTOUSH

SERVES 2–4

★

1 small cauliflower,
    cut into bite-sized florets
3 tablespoons olive oil,
    plus extra for the cauliflower
juice of 1 lemon
300g mixed cherry tomatoes
½ red onion, finely sliced
1 small garlic clove,
    finely chopped
1 tablespoon red wine vinegar
2 mini summer cucumbers
1 small Little Gem lettuce
2 pitta breads
leaves from a small bunch
    of parsley, roughly chopped
leaves from a small bunch
    of mint, roughly chopped
1 teaspoon sumac
salt and pepper

There are loads of riffs on bread salads, from the croutons in a Caesar salad to the torn loaf in an Italian panzanella. This is a Middle Eastern version, made with lots of fresh veg and toasted pitta bread, with the sharp tang of lemon juice and citrusy sumac, and handfuls of fresh herbs.

Preheat your oven to 200°C (Gas Mark 6). Place the cauliflower florets in a roasting tin. Oil them well and season with salt, pepper and a good squeeze of lemon juice. Roast for 12–15 minutes, until nicely coloured and tender. Leave to cool for 5 minutes.

Meanwhile, cut the tomatoes into an interesting mix of wedges and slices. Put them in a mixing bowl, along with the onion, garlic, vinegar and 3 tablespoons of olive oil. Season with salt and pepper. Gently mix together and leave to macerate.

Halve the cucumbers lengthways. Remove the soft seedy cores with the tip of a teaspoon. Cut into 1cm angled slices. Cut the root away from the lettuce and break it into individual leaves. Keep the small leaves whole, tear the larger ones in half.

Toast the pitta breads or place them in the oven after the cauliflower, until toasted and crisp. Tear them into bite-sized pieces.

Throw the cauliflower, cucumber, lettuce leaves, torn pittas, herbs and half the sumac into the mixing bowl and toss everything together. Taste and adjust the seasoning with salt, pepper and lemon juice. Pile on to plates and sprinkle with the rest of the sumac.

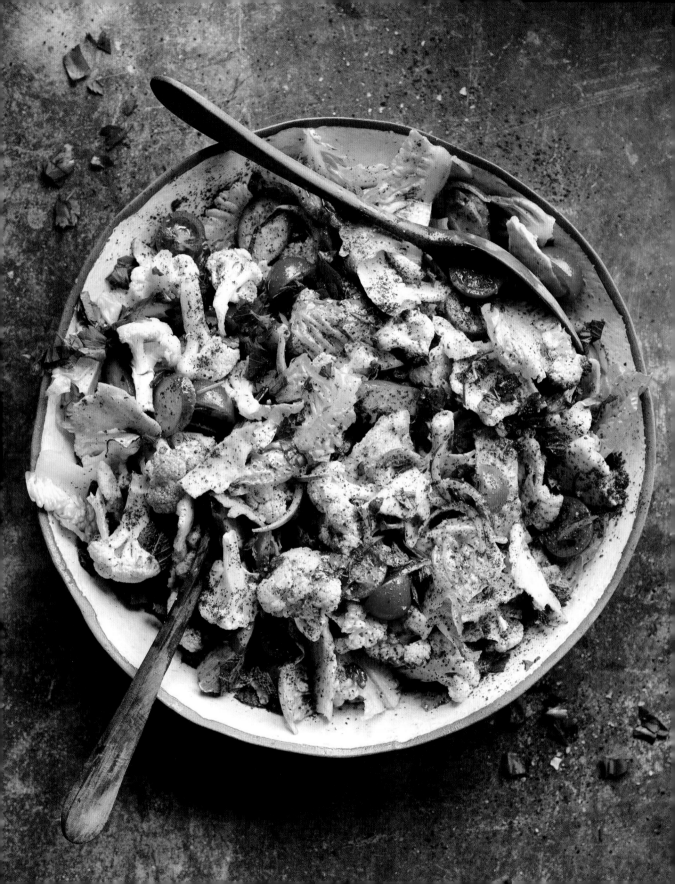

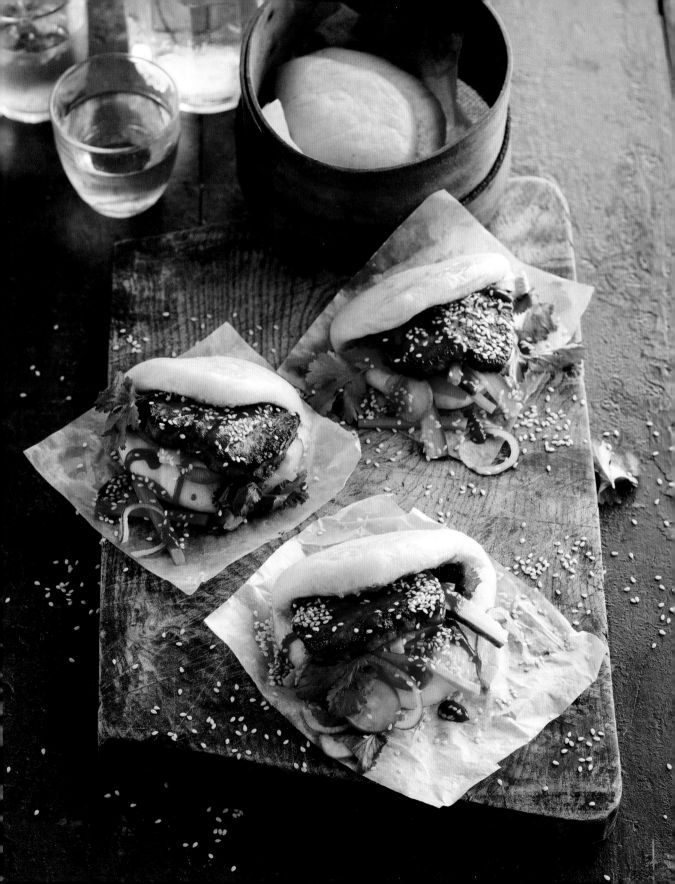

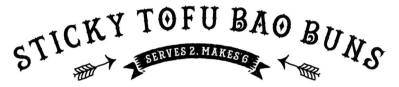

STICKY TOFU BAO BUNS
SERVES 2, MAKES 6

For the tofu
2cm piece of fresh root ginger,
   finely grated
1 garlic clove, finely chopped
2 tablespoons rice wine
2 tablespoons soy sauce
2 tablespoons agave syrup
1 teaspoon Chinese five spice
300g firm tofu
2 tablespoons flavourless
   vegetable oil

For the buns
80ml warm water
40ml unsweetened rice
   or oat milk
1 teaspoon vegetable oil,
   plus extra for brushing
1 teaspoon sugar
1 teaspoon fast-action
   dried yeast
200g plain flour,
   plus extra for dusting
½ teaspoon baking powder
¼ teaspoon salt

To serve
pickled veg (see page 100)
leaves from a small bunch
   of coriander
½ tablespoon sesame seeds
sriracha sauce (optional)

These steamed buns are light, fluffy and addictive. Six buns feels about right for two... maybe a bit indulgent, but you'll find that two is not enough, so best err on the side of caution. I'd probably eat all six!

Start with the tofu. Mix everything except the tofu and oil in a shallow bowl to make a marinade. Cut the tofu into 6 equal slabs and turn them in the marinade. Leave to marinate while you continue.

To make the bun dough, mix the warm water, milk, oil, sugar and yeast together in a bowl. Leave for 15 minutes, until the liquid looks foamy and active. Add the flour, baking powder and salt. Knead for 10 minutes with your hands, or in a food mixer fitted with a dough hook, or until glossy and elastic. Form into a ball and cover the bowl with clingfilm. Leave somewhere warm until doubled in size, this may take a couple of hours.

When the dough has risen, turn it out on to a floured work surface and knock the air out of it. Divide into 6 equal pieces and shape into balls. Roll each ball out into an oval and brush the tops lightly with oil. Place a chopstick in the middle of an oval, widthways, and fold the dough gently in half. Slide the chopstick out and place the bun on a small square of baking parchment. Repeat to shape all 6 buns. Loosely cover with clingfilm and wait until they have doubled in size again, which should take 30 minutes to an hour.

Recipe continues overleaf

When they are ready, place them in a steamer, on their parchment squares, and steam for 12–15 minutes until light and risen. This might be easier in batches, unless you have more than one steamer. The buns will last well for a few hours and you can reheat them by steaming again for a couple of minutes.

To cook the tofu, heat the oil in a frying pan. Scrape as much of the marinade off the tofu slices as you can, so they will brown (but reserve the marinade). Fry them for 2–3 minutes a side, until golden. Tip the marinade into the pan and let it bubble away for a minute or so until thick and sticky, turning the tofu to coat it.

Tease open the steamed buns along the line left by the chopstick and place a slice of tofu in the middle of each, along with any marinade left in the pan. Add some pickles, some torn coriander leaves and a sprinkling of sesame seeds. If you want some heat, add a streak of sriracha to finish.

ROCKING CAULI and BANGING BROCCOLI

SERVES 4

2 tablespoons olive oil
2 tablespoons toasted sesame oil
1 garlic clove, finely grated
30g fresh root ginger,
    finely grated
2 tablespoons balsamic vinegar
1 teaspoon wholegrain mustard
1 teaspoon soy sauce
1 teaspoon maple syrup
juice of ½ lemon, or to taste
1 head of broccoli
1 cauliflower
pepper

I'm terrible for reaching for the crisps, so I came up with this recipe for a good-for-you snack when you're feeling peckish. I love these little tasty mouthfuls of sweet-and-sour goodness. The problem is, as soon as you've eaten one, the rest follow. Before you know it... all gone. This also makes a good side dish, or you could mix in some noodles for a healthy meal.

Get a good-sized jam jar with a lid and put in everything except the broccoli and cauli. Shake it like Bez's maracas until all the dressing's all emulsified. Taste and adjust the seasoning with pepper or lemon juice, as you prefer.

Break up the broccoli and the cauliflower into florets and stick into a saucepan of boiling water for no more than 3–4 minutes, to make sure the veg still has a good crunch to it. The last thing you need is soggy veg! (You can use a steamer if you prefer.)

Drain, then return all the florets to the saucepan. Pour over as little or as much of the dressing as you want and mix everything together.

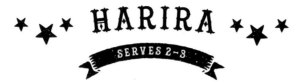

HARIRA

SERVES 2–3

2 tablespoons olive oil
1 onion, finely chopped
1 celery stick, finely chopped
1 carrot, finely chopped
1 garlic clove, finely chopped
2cm piece of fresh root ginger,
   finely grated
1 teaspoon ground cumin
½ teaspoon smoked paprika
½ cinnamon stick
small pinch of saffron threads
   (optional, see recipe
   introduction)
1 tablespoon harissa
½ x 400g can chickpeas, drained
30g red lentils, rinsed
30g basmati rice, rinsed
200g tomato passata
700ml vegetable stock
   (for homemade, see page 121)
salt and pepper
juice of 1 lemon
leaves from a small bunch
   of coriander, chopped

This is a real winter warmer of a soup and packed with protein on all fronts, as the original recipe was designed as the ideal food with which to break a long fast. The saffron isn't necessary, but adds a special something. If you don't have any, ½ teaspoon ground turmeric can give an approximation of its colour, although not its taste.

Warm the oil in a large saucepan over a gentle heat. Gently cook the onion, celery and carrot for 10 minutes, until starting to soften.

Add the garlic, ginger, spices and harissa. Cook for 2 more minutes before tipping in the chickpeas, lentils, rice, passata and stock. Bring to the boil, then reduce the heat to a simmer, season with salt and pepper and cook gently until everything is cooked and softened. (This should take about 25 minutes.)

Taste and tweak the seasoning with salt, pepper and a squeeze or so of lemon juice, to your liking. Divide between deep warm bowls and sprinkle with coriander.

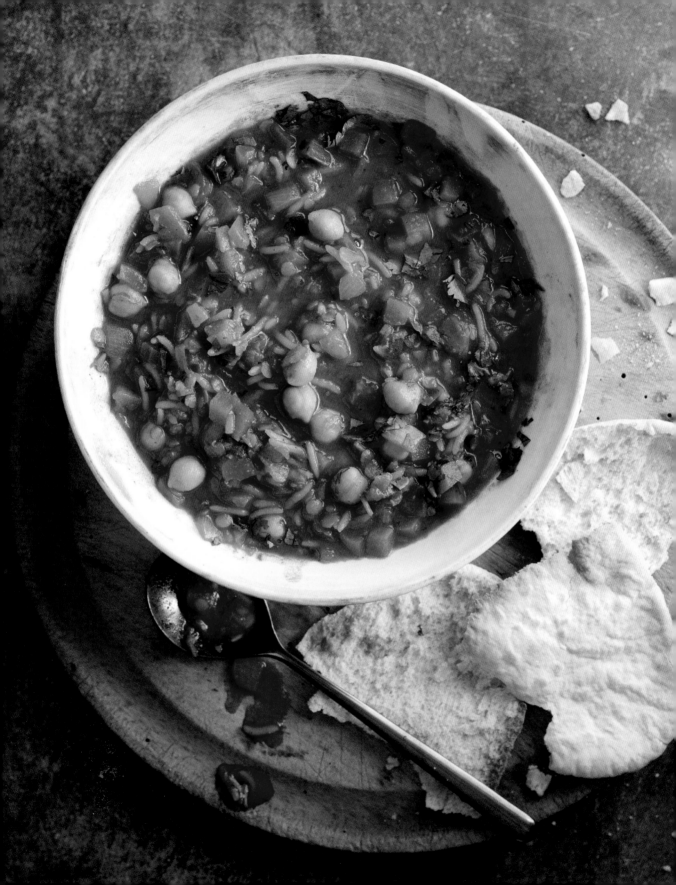

SALAD SOUP WITH WILD GARLIC PESTO

SERVES 2

2 tablespoons olive oil
4 spring onions, sliced
200g new potatoes,
    peeled and finely chopped
1 bay leaf
700ml light vegetable stock
    (for homemade, see page 121)
2 small Little Gem lettuces,
    or ½ round lettuce such as
    Butterhead, shredded
200g frozen peas
leaves from a small bunch
    of parsley
4–5 mint leaves
3 tablespoons vegan crème
    fraîche (optional)
salt and pepper

For the pesto
50g wild garlic
30g toasted pine nuts
20g toasted almonds
2 tablespoons nutritional yeast
4 tablespoons olive oil
juice of 1 lemon

Don't be put off by lettuce in a soup, the whole point of this dish is to be fresh and green! Wild garlic is a native British leaf that grows abundantly on countryside verges and in woodland from March to May. It has a proper garlicky poke to it. Some veg box companies sell it. If the season has passed, you can replace it with basil to make a more classic pesto.

Warm the olive oil in a large saucepan. Gently fry the spring onions for 5 minutes, until starting to soften. Add the potatoes and bay leaf. Cook gently for a further 2 minutes, then tip in the stock. Season with salt, bring to the boil, then reduce the heat to a simmer and cook for 10 minutes.

Meanwhile, make the pesto by blitzing the wild garlic, pine nuts, almonds, nutritional yeast and oil together in a food processor. (You can also make it in a mortar and pestle, with a little patience and muscle power.) Season with salt and a squeeze or two of lemon juice, to taste.

Add the lettuce and peas to the saucepan and cook for a further 7–8 minutes, until the potatoes are completely soft. Remove the bay leaf, then tear in the parsley and mint leaves and grind in some black pepper. Blend the soup until completely smooth, adding a dash more hot water if it seems a bit thick.

Taste and tweak the seasoning. Divide between deep warm bowls and add a swirl of vegan crème fraîche, if you like. Finish each bowl with a generous blob of pesto.

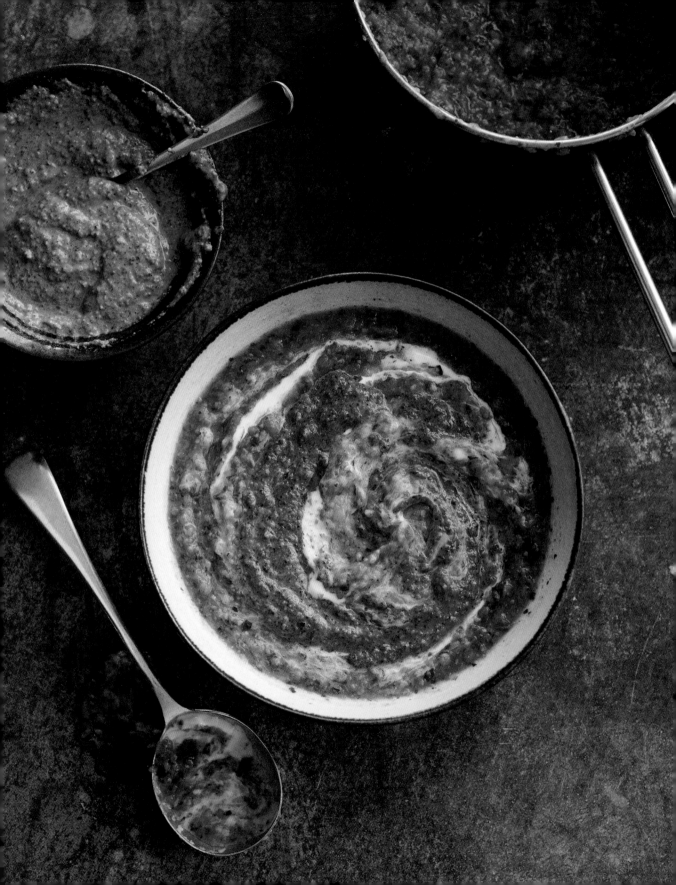

ROAST BEETROOT and SMOKED TOFU SALAD

SERVES 2

6 beetroots
small bunch of thyme
splash of olive oil
handful of kale,
   coarse stalks removed
1 tablespoon maple syrup
200g pack smoked firm tofu,
   cut into cubes
handful of walnuts
1 quantity Pritchard's dressing
   (optional, see page 118)
salt and pepper

Beets appear in my diet at least five times a week, as I always have beet juice in my morning smoothie after my gym sesh. Roast beets are so good compared to the boiled version. I think, to many, beetroots are like Marmite: you either love 'em or hate 'em, but trust me, if you roast them they taste so much better... especially with a little coating of maple syrup. Add the smoked tofu, kale and walnuts and you've got a nutritious, tasty salad.

Preheat the oven to 200°C (Gas Mark 6).

Cut the beetroot into quarters and chuck it in a roasting tin. Sprinkle over some fresh thyme – I find if you grab a bunch of thyme and rub it between your hands, the leaves fall off in a nice sprinkle. Drizzle over the oil and place in the oven for 30 minutes.

While the beets are roasting, cook the kale by boiling it in plenty of salted water for 3–4 minutes. Kale can be quite tough, so take a bit out and nibble it to make sure it is tender. Drain.

After 30 minutes, take the beets out of the oven and reduce the oven temperature to 180°C (Gas Mark 4). Drizzle over the maple syrup, mix around until all the pieces of beetroot are evenly coated and return to the oven for 10 minutes.

Take the beets out of the oven and mix in the kale, tofu and walnuts. Toss and serve up. Dress with the Pritchard's dressing, or serve as it is. Either way, it's amazing!

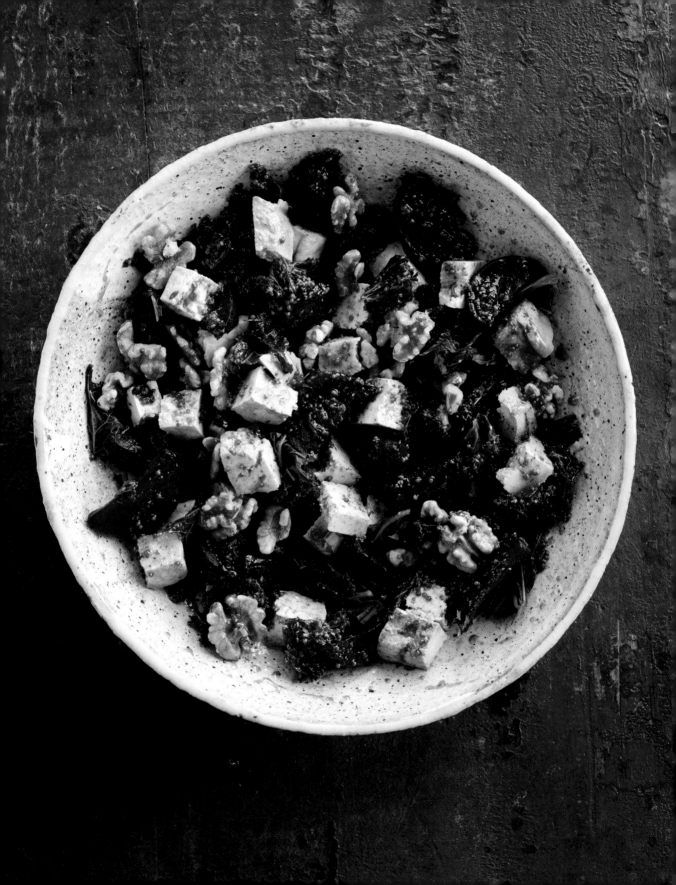

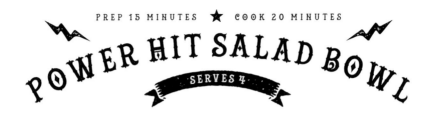

POWER HIT SALAD BOWL

SERVES 4

12 new potatoes
200g frozen edamame beans
200g canned chickpeas
   (drained weight),
   liquid reserved
your choice of dressing
   (see below)
200g baby spinach
200g rocket or watercress,
   coarse stalks removed
250g good-quality tomatoes,
   chopped
4 spring onions, finely chopped
2 avocados, pitted and sliced
handful of peanuts

Smoked paprika dressing
2 tablespoons olive oil
1 tablespoon white wine vinegar
1 teaspoon Dijon mustard
juice of ½ lemon
½ garlic clove, finely grated
1 teaspoon smoked paprika
1 teaspoon maple syrup
salt and pepper

Pritchard's dressing
2 tablespoons olive oil
1 tablespoon toasted sesame oil
1½ tablespoons balsamic vinegar
½ garlic clove, finely grated
juice of ½ lemon
1 teaspoon maple syrup
1 teaspoon wholegrain mustard
salt and pepper

Caesar dressing: **see page 52**

I love when spring hits and shop shelves are groaning with fresh green produce. It's my fave time of the year, as the weather's getting better for my bike rides! I need something full of goodness to eat, so I make myself this. I've included chickpeas and edamame for a proper protein hit. For the new potatoes, use Jersey Royals or Pembrokeshire News if you can, but no biggy if not.

Bring 2 saucepans of salted water to the boil. In the first, cook the potatoes for 15–20 minutes and, in the other pan, cook the frozen edamame for 5 minutes. Drain both when they're ready.

While they cook, drain the chickpeas (retain the liquid to make mayonnaise or meringue in another recipe). Make your choice of dressing: keep an empty jam jar or something similar in the cupboard for mixing dressings and simply tip all the ingredients in. To emulsify the dressings, it helps if you're playing some heavy metal in the background: just rock out to Motorhead with the jar in your hand and it'll mix up just fine.

Get a big salad bowl, tip in the spinach and rocket or watercress and add the tomatoes, spring onions, chickpeas, peanuts and drained edamame beans and potatoes. Layer on the avocados. Forget the salad tongs, just get those hands in (making sure they are clean of course).

Add your chosen dressing and serve straight away, as you don't want the leaves to get soggy.

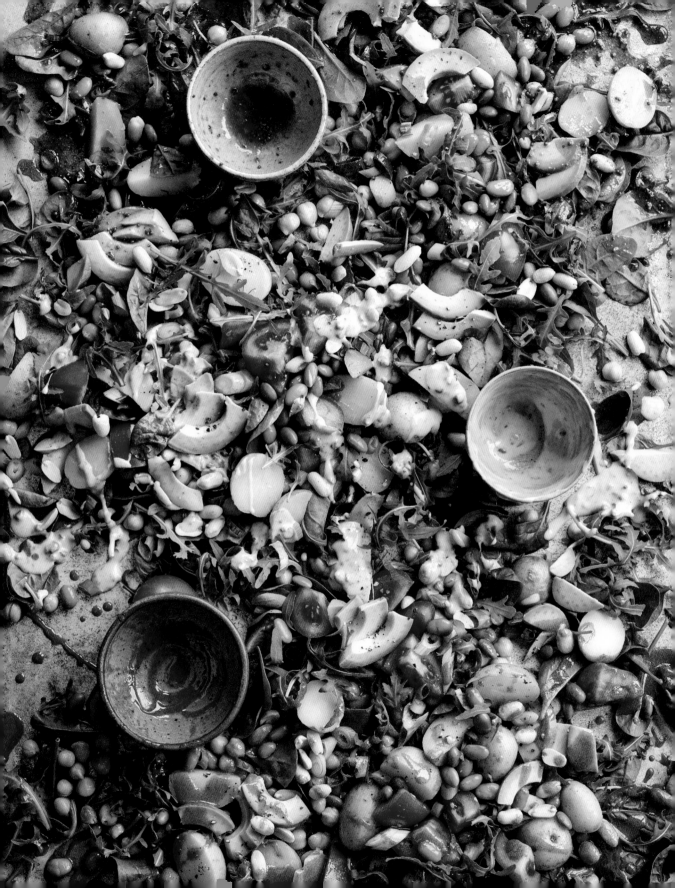

SMOKEY, POKEY SWEETCORN and SPINACH CHOWDER

SERVES 2

2 tablespoons olive oil
1 carrot, finely chopped
2 celery sticks, finely chopped
1 leek, finely sliced
1 potato, finely chopped
sweetcorn kernels from
    2 sweetcorn cobs, or 250g
    canned sweetcorn
2 garlic cloves, finely chopped
1 teaspoon thyme leaves
1 bay leaf
pinch of chilli flakes
125ml white wine
600ml light vegetable stock,
    preferably made with
    sweetcorn (see page 121)
100ml unsweetened oat
    or almond milk
80g baby spinach
½ tablespoon liquid smoke
    (optional)
small bunch of chives
salt and pepper

It is easy to remove the kernels from a fresh corn cob. Simply discard the outer husks, slice the broadest end off to make a flat base and stand the cob upright on a chopping board. Run a sharp knife down the sides and the kernels will come cascading off. The empty cobs make a welcome addition to a stock pot, especially if the stock is destined for the chowder itself; a virtuous and thrifty circle. Liquid smoke (widely available in supermarkets and online) is a nice addition, but not vital; you could get a similar result with a pinch of smoked paprika sprinkled on each bowl at the end.

Warm the olive oil in a large saucepan. Gently fry the carrot and celery for 5 minutes, until starting to soften. Add the leek, potato, sweetcorn, garlic, thyme, bay and chilli. Cook gently for a further 5 minutes, stirring often.

Tip in the wine and increase the heat. Let the liquid reduce until it has almost disappeared, then tip in the stock and season with salt and pepper. Bring to the boil, then reduce the heat to a gentle simmer and cook for 20 minutes, until everything is tender.

Add the milk to the pan and return the chowder to a simmer. Remove the bay leaf. Transfer one-third of the soup to a food processer or blender and blitz until smooth. Return it to the pan and stir in the spinach until wilted, just for a minute or so. Stir in the liquid smoke (if using). Season to taste.

Serve in deep warm bowls with a few chives snipped over the top.

BONELESS BROTH THREE WAYS

MAKES 1 LITRE

★

2 onions, skins left on,
    roughly chopped
2 carrots,
    roughly chopped
3 celery sticks,
    roughly chopped
1 garlic clove, split open
small bunch of parsley
3–4 thyme sprigs
10 black peppercorns
2 bay leaves
1.2 litres water

OPTIONAL EXTRAS

Leek tops
Similar to onions in flavour,
so consider using half leeks
and half onions.

Mushrooms
These add a deep, earthy, savoury
flavour. Simply crumble some
dried mushrooms in with the veg:
10–15g will be enough, as a little
goes a long way.

Sweetcorn cobs
They add a nice comforting
sweetness.

Tomatoes
These can add a savoury, umami
flavour, much like 'shrooms do.
Don't go overboard; 2 sliced
tomatoes should do.

A good veg stock is infinitely useful, so it is worth making a big batch. Plus, it freezes well. Ideally your stock pot should be populated by surplus veg and trimmings, so that you aren't using up your premium veg; most busy kitchens keep a scrap-pot for stock – a home for all the onion ends, leek tops, bendy carrots and parsley stalks.

THE BASIC BLEND

Place everything in a large saucepan and bring to a very gentle simmer. Cook for 45 minutes, making sure it stays on a low simmer and doesn't start a rolling boil. Remove from the heat and allow to sit for 30 minutes to allow the flavours to develop further, before straining through a sieve.

QUICK AND LIGHT

You can halve the cooking time of your stock by coarsely grating all the veg before adding it to the pan. This increases the surface area and draws the flavour out faster. Simmer for 20 minutes and strain immediately – any longer and you run the risk of it turning into a mushy soup.

DARK AND ROASTED

This is more involved, but produces a darker, more complex stock. You want to get some colour on the veg before adding it to the water, as all the golden edges add deeper flavours and a dark caramel colour. Toss with oil and roast for 25–30 minutes at 200°C (Gas Mark 6) until nicely coloured and almost burnt at the edges – the onions in particular. Tip them into a saucepan with everything else and follow the instructions for the basic stock.

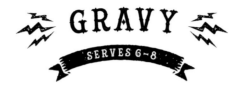

GRAVY

SERVES 6–8

125ml white wine
1 litre dark vegetable stock
(see page 121)
1 tablespoon nutritional yeast
2 teaspoons brown rice miso
2 tablespoons cornflour,
or to taste
red wine vinegar,
to taste (optional)
salt and pepper

The proper destiny of a stock has to be a gravy. Dark and roasted stock is the ideal base, with some dried mushrooms and a couple of tomatoes added to boost the umami flavour. If the stock is good enough, the gravy will just need the sharpness of the wine and a little nudge from the yeast and miso. If you are using this recipe at Christmas, try switching the white wine for red, or even using a snifter of port instead.

Place a saucepan over a medium heat and add the wine. Let it boil down until reduced by half.

Add the stock, yeast and miso. Bring to the boil, stirring as you do, then reduce the heat to a gentle simmer.

Mix the cornflour with a dash of cold water to form a paste. Stir it into the gravy and return it to the boil, stirring, until thickened. (Use more cornflour if you like a thicker gravy.) Taste and season with salt and pepper. If you think it needs a touch more acidity, you can add a small dash of red wine vinegar to your liking.

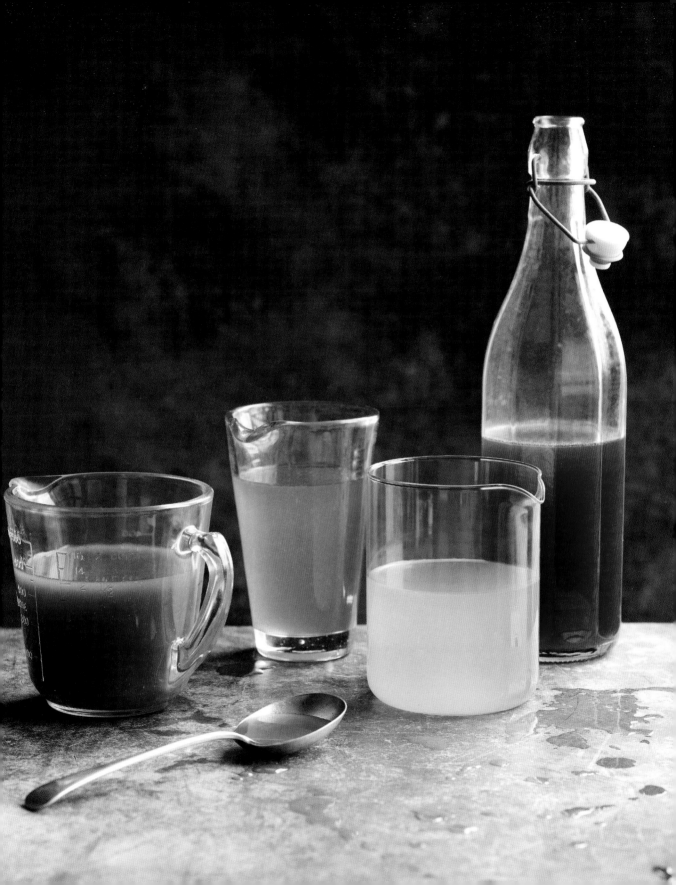

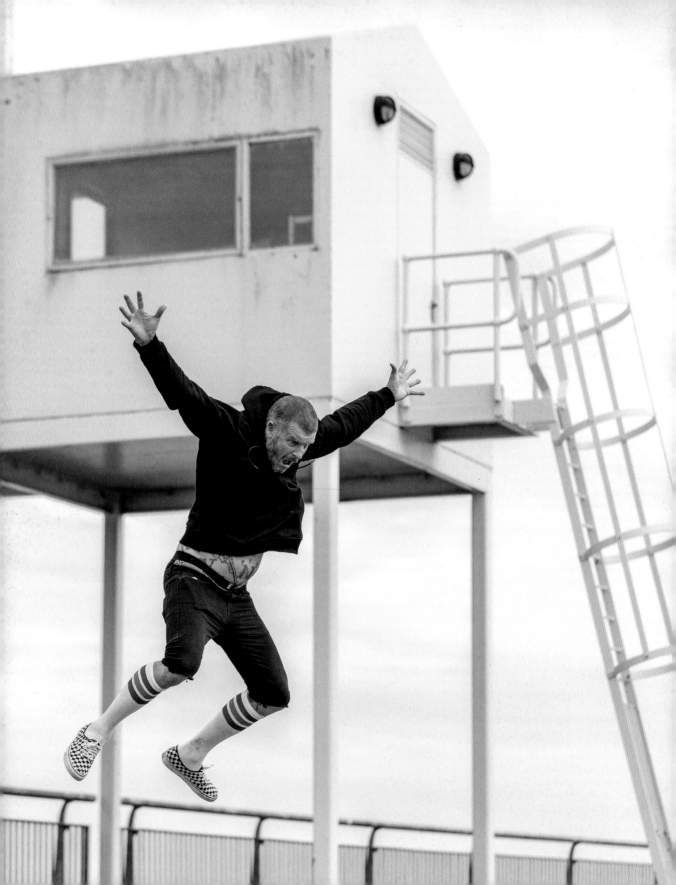

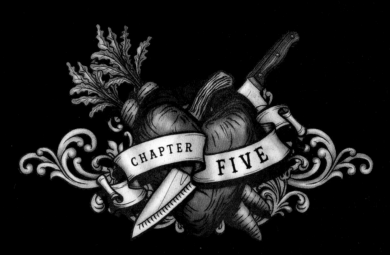

CHAPTER FIVE

SWEET STUFF

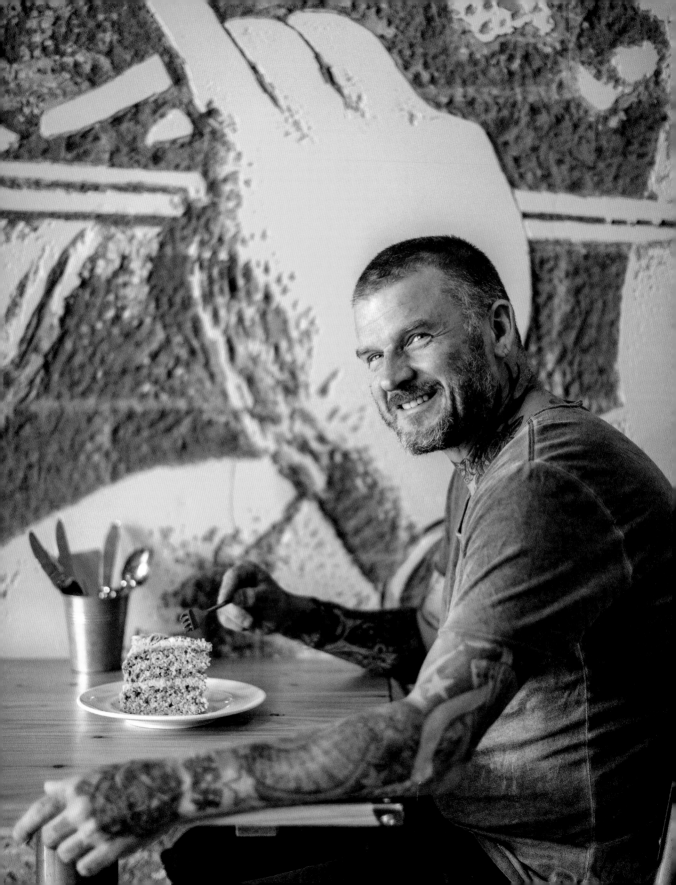

At a restaurant, if I have eaten a great starter and main course but the puddings are a let-down, I'm gutted. I want that beauty to be put in front of me, then for everyone at the table to silently compare their pud to mine and decide who has the best. Be honest now, we all do it! If someone has a better-looking dessert than yours, you instantly either want to send yours back... or get a taste of theirs. Or do what my fiancée does: turn down a pudding, then steal mine!

When I went vegan, I had the classic vegan baking problem: what was I gonna use as an egg substitute? When, in the first series of *Dirty Vegan*, the Women's Institute set me the challenge of baking vegan cakes for them, I instantly headed to Naturally Kind foods in Bridgend, where Andy and Sarah bake the best vegan cakes I've tasted. There are many ways of substituting eggs in cakes: chia seeds, flax seeds, nut butter, tofu, bicarbonate of soda and vinegar... and, of course, aquafaba (the liquid from a can of chickpeas). Andy and Sarah really helped advise me on my baking... and the WI loved the chocolate cupcakes I came up with.

I very much enjoyed spending time with my ladies at the Institute, they were so much fun and really welcoming. I'll visit them again very soon for a catch-up – over some tea and vegan cake, of course!

There's a recipe in this chapter that handed me a great deal of failures before I finally got it right. It was the one for my fave pud before I became a vegan: panna cotta. I can't use gelatine any more, so I used agar agar, which comes from a type of algae. After about 10 puddly failures, I asked my friend Laura from Tidy Kitchen for advice... and the result is banging! I wanted to add my own little pzazz to the recipe, so I experimented with oat and coconut cream together and came up with a beauty of a panna cotta, that I hope you all enjoy too.

As far as vegan cream is concerned, you can't go far wrong with sweetened coconut cream. It's so tasty and, when you add vanilla, it is the perfect substitute for dairy cream in my eyes. Dollop it on sticky toffee pudding and I guarantee you'll be picking up the plate and licking it all off... table manners right outta the window!

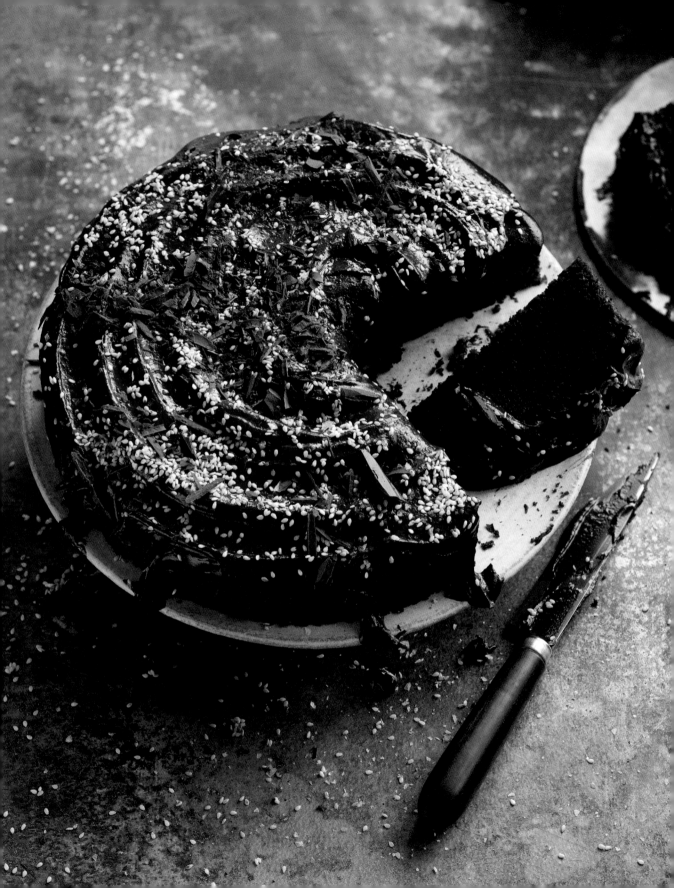

GUEST CHEF: CHOCOLATE ORANGE CHIFFON CAKE

SERVES 8–10

For the cake

130g deodorized coconut oil, melted, plus extra for the tin

310g plain flour

10g cornflour

100g cocoa powder

1 teaspoon bicarbonate of soda

1½ teaspoons baking powder

1½ teaspoons fine sea salt

375g caster sugar

3 teaspoons vanilla extract

1 teaspoon cider vinegar

40g light tahini

finely grated zest of 2 oranges

200ml unsweetened non-dairy milk

250ml strongly brewed coffee (decaf, if you so desire)

125g aquafaba (the liquid from a can of chickpeas), chilled

½ lemon

⅛ teaspoon cream of tartar

For the ganache

120g vegan dark chocolate, finely chopped

30g cocoa powder, sifted

40g light tahini

finely grated zest and juice of 1 orange

60g maple syrup

120ml unsweetened non-dairy milk

60g deodorized coconut oil

2 teaspoons vanilla extract

1½ teaspoons sea salt flakes

This show-stopping number is by Kelsey of Vanderstarre Cakes in Devon, who deserves a spot in this book for her plant-based cake mastery. She spent months creating and testing this and was at her wit's end, as it kept collapsing… only to discover one of the heating elements in her oven had broken! She thought she was losing her baking mojo, but it's all good. And this cake is – only one way to describe it – proper banging! Truly worthy of a celebration. Kelsey always uses cake strips for her cakes, which are easy to find online and produce deliciously moist sponge layers. (Cakes with dry edges? Get outta here.) Just soak them in water while you prep your cake batter, then wrap them around your prepared baking tins. Seriously guys, this is not a drill, these strips are magic.

Slide the oven rack into the middle of the oven and preheat it to 160°C (Gas Mark 3). Lightly grease a 23cm springform cake tin with oil and line the bottom with baking parchment.

In a large bowl, sift together the flour, cornflour, cocoa powder, bicarbonate of soda, baking powder and salt.

In a separate bowl, whisk 250g of the caster sugar with the melted coconut oil, vanilla, cider vinegar, tahini, orange zest, milk and coffee.

Recipe continues overleaf

To decorate
10g sesame seeds, toasted
sea salt flakes (optional)
vegan dark chocolate shavings
(optional)

DECORATING OPTIONS

Either
The ganache can be poured
luxuriously over the cooled
cake, then sprinkled with toasted
sesame seeds and sea salt flakes
for an indulgent looking finish.

Or
Leave the ganache to chill in
the fridge for 20–30 minutes
until spreadable, then use it to
generously frost your chiffon cake.
Sprinkle with toasted sesame
seeds and chocolate shavings.

Now you need to whisk the aquafaba. This is best done in a
stand mixer fitted with the whisk attachment, or in a large bowl
using a hand-held electric mixer. Prepare the bowl by wiping
the inside with a halved lemon; this is to remove any traces
of fat, which will stop the aquafaba whisking to full volume.

Combine the chilled aquafaba with the cream of tartar and
start whisking on medium speed for 2 minutes until frothy.
With the mixer still running, slowly add the remaining 125g
caster sugar, 1 tablespoon at a time, allowing the sugar to
incorporate before adding the next tablespoon. Continue
whisking for 8–10 minutes, until the aquafaba has trebled in
volume and miraculously transformed into fluffy meringue.
Stop the mixer.

Pour the liquid coconut oil mixture into the dry flour mixture
and whisk together until just combined. You should have
a rich chocolate batter with only the odd streak of flour.
The less whisking you can manage here, the better.

Now add one-third of the aquafaba meringue and gently
fold it in to loosen the mixture. This must be done gently in
order to incorporate as much air as possible into your cake.
Add half the remaining meringue and fold in gently but
firmly, until everything is just incorporated. Finish with
the remaining meringue, folding until you're left with
a light and airy chocolate mixture. Do not overmix.

Apply cake strips to your prepared tin. Without delay, pour
the batter into the tin and bake for 55–70 minutes, or until a
toothpick inserted in the centre of the cake comes out clean
and the sponge springs lightly back when gently prodded.
Cool completely before removing from the tin.

For the ganache, put the chocolate, cocoa powder, tahini,
orange zest and juice and maple syrup in a large heatproof
bowl. Heat the non-dairy milk and coconut oil in a small
saucepan to just under the boil, swirling gently to evenly
distribute the heat, before pouring it over the chocolate
mixture. Leave, without stirring, for a minute or 2. Whisk
until silky smooth, then whisk in the vanilla and salt.

Decorate the cake choosing one of the options above!

CHOCOLATE AVO MOUSSE

SERVES 2 GENEROUSLY

3 ripe medium avocados
2 tablespoons cocoa powder
1 tablespoon vanilla extract
4 tablespoons maple syrup,
   or to taste
250ml oat cream
800g vegan 85% cocoa solids
   chocolate (you can use 70%,
   if that's all you can find), plus
   grated chocolate to serve
raspberries, to serve

Who doesn't like a choccie mousse? This one is full of the good fats from avocados. Avocados as a pudding? Yep, it tastes brilliant, trust me. Give it a go and enjoy every spoonful.

Remove and discard the skins and stones from the avocados and place the flesh into a blender with the cocoa powder, vanilla extract, maple syrup and oat cream and blend until smooth.

Put a saucepan of water on the hob and place a heatproof bowl on top; the base of the bowl should not touch the water. Break the chocolate into pieces in the bowl and let the heat of the water slowly melt the chocolate. Once the chocolate's melted, add it to the avocado mix and stir it all together until you're left with a lovely smooth chocolaty mousse.

Taste and, if it needs a little more sweetness, add a little more maple syrup... I find this amount of syrup just perfect, but of course we're all different.

Put it in the fridge to chill for an hour or so, then grate over some chocolate, scatter on some raspberries and enjoy!

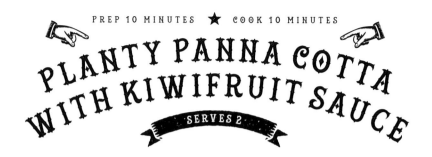

PLANTY PANNA COTTA WITH KIWIFRUIT SAUCE

SERVES 2

For the panna cotta
160ml coconut cream
250ml oat cream
1 teaspoon agar agar powder
1 teaspoon vanilla bean paste
2 tablespoons maple syrup
   or agave syrup
a little flavourless oil
a few mint leaves,
   to serve (optional)

For the kiwi sauce
2 ripe kiwifruits,
   cut into thin slices
1 tablespoon maple syrup
1 tablespoon water

Before I was vegan, I was a massive fan of panna cotta. I used to love seeing it turn up in front of me with that slight wobble and look forward to sticking my spoon into it. This recipe has taken me ages to sort out – along the way I've had many puddles of pud when I removed the moulds – but I got it right in the end!

Put all the ingredients for the panna cottas – except the oil and mint – in a saucepan, place it over a medium-low heat and bring to a simmer.

Lightly oil 2 ramekins with flavourless oil. Pour the cream mixture in, cover and put in the fridge to set for 3–4 hours.

Keeping some kiwi slices aside for decoration, put the rest in a saucepan with the maple syrup and measured water. Place over a medium heat and bring to a simmer, to soften the kiwifruits. Pulse in a blender until combined. Place a sieve over a bowl and pour the kiwifruit mixture in, leaving all the pulp behind in the sieve. Loosen the sauce in the bowl with a little extra water if it looks too thick.

Run a knife around the edges of the ramekins and the panna cottas should plop out on to plates. If not, scream and shout at them for a bit – that should help. It made me feel better when I kept getting the recipe wrong!

Pour the sauce around the panna cottas. Use the reserved kiwifruits to decorate as well as a bit of mint, if you have any knocking around.

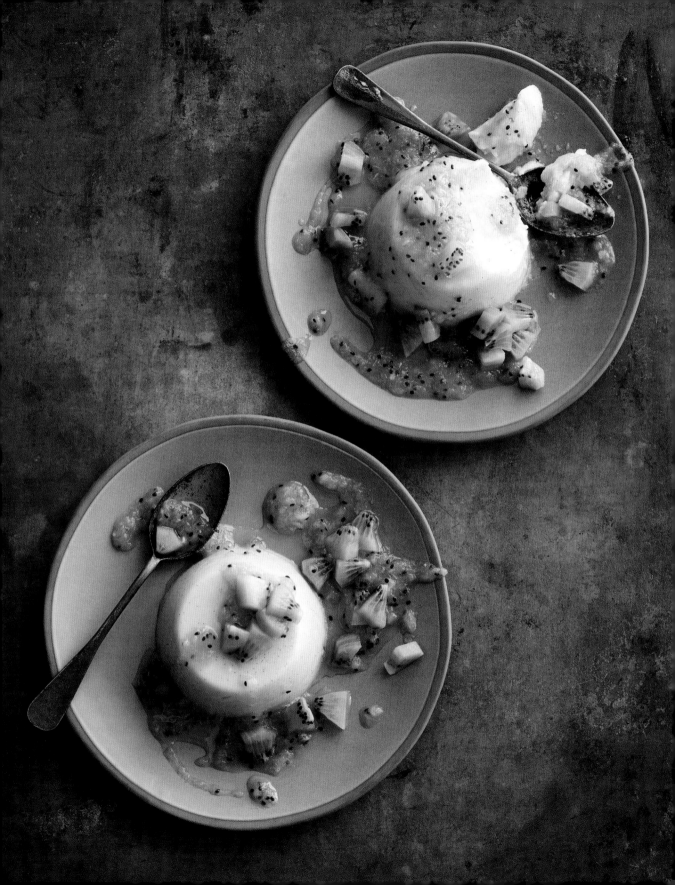

CHOCOLATE CINDER TOFFEE

MAKES 12–16 PIECES

6 tbsp golden syrup
200g caster sugar
2 teaspoons bicarbonate of soda
100g vegan dark chocolate
sea salt flakes (optional)

Also known as honeycomb or hokey pokey, this is basically a homemade version of a Crunchie bar. It feels a bit like a science experiment when the bicarb turns the sugar into a foam. Anything involving hot sugar is properly dangerous, so have a good pair of oven gloves to hand. This recipe does rely on getting the sugar to an ideal temperature; you can attempt to do it by timing or by eye, but without practice it can be hit and miss. A sugar thermometer is your best bet.

Line a baking tin with baking parchment. Place the syrup and sugar in a high-sided saucepan and warm them over a gentle heat. Stir occasionally, to help the sugar dissolve into the syrup. When it is all liquid, stop stirring and increase the heat until it reaches 145°C, this will take about 10 minutes.

Remove the pan from the heat and stir in the bicarbonate of soda with a wooden spoon. It will start to foam and rise in the pan. A few good stirs are enough, you don't want to knock too much air out of the mixture. Immediately tip the mixture into the prepared tin. Leave to cool completely.

Break the chocolate into small pieces and place it in a heatproof bowl. Sit the bowl above a pan of simmering water until the chocolate has melted (make sure the base of the bowl does not touch the water).

Break the cinder toffee into pieces. Dip the ends into the melted chocolate and place on a wire rack to cool. If you are feeling a bit hipster, add a pinch of sea salt flakes before the chocolate has set. You can store the pieces in an airtight container, where they should last for a few days before they start to soften... but you're unlikely get to that stage.

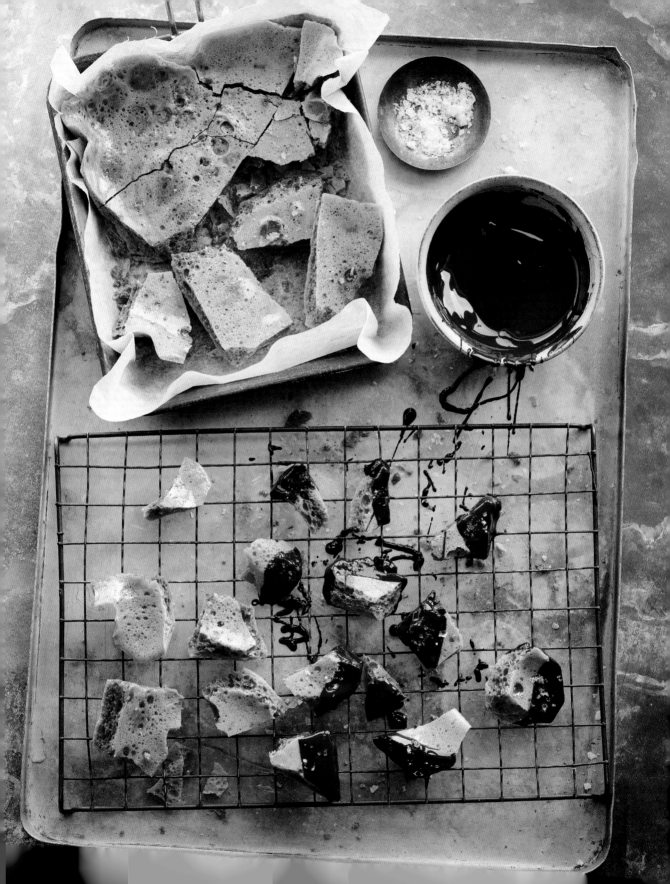

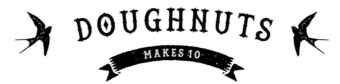

DOUGHNUTS

MAKES 10

125ml unsweetened oat milk
5g sachet fast-action dried yeast
25g caster sugar, plus extra
　for dusting
30g deodorized coconut oil
60ml aquafaba (the liquid
　from a can of chickpeas)
250g white bread flour,
　plus extra for dusting
5g fine sea salt
about 1.5 litres sunflower or
　vegetable oil, for deep-frying

I'll say it straight off: good doughnuts are a faff to make. They need a bit of bread-making skill, as well as time, patience and a light touch, but they are worth the labour. Be prepared to deep-fry, and you'll need a cooking thermometer to keep an eye on the oil temperature.

Gently warm the oat milk in a saucepan, but don't boil it, you want it like a warm bath. Pour into a jug and add the yeast and sugar. Mix well and set aside for 10 minutes. This helps to activate the yeast.

Add the oil to the warm milk, until melted, then pour in the aquafaba and mix together.

Sift the flour into a food mixer bowl and tip in the milk mixture. Use a dough hook to mix it on a medium speed for 4 minutes. Leave to rest for 15 minutes.

Add the salt to the dough and mix on a medium speed for a further 5 minutes. The dough should be glossy and feel quite elastic and sticky. Shape it into a rough ball, cover the bowl with clingfilm and leave somewhere warm until doubled in size, 1–2 hours.

Knock the dough back (just punch it lightly), cover once more and and pop it into the fridge for 20 mins. (The dough is easier to shape and handle when chilled.)

The next day, line a large baking sheet or chopping board with baking parchment. Lightly dust your work surface with flour and scrape out the dough. Divide into 10 equal balls, about 50g each. Working fast before they get too warm, shape and roll each piece into a firm bun shape. Place them on the baking parchment, with plenty of room in between to allow them to rise. Cover lightly with clingfilm and leave somewhere warm until doubled in size.

When they have risen, pop them in the fridge for 20 minutes while you get the oil ready, it makes them easier to handle. (It may be easier to tease them off the baking parchment with a spatula when you need them.)

Get a heavy, deep-sided saucepan and add the oil until 6–8cm deep, you don't want it to be more than one-third full for safety reasons. Place over a medium heat and slowly bring the oil up to 180°C.

Fill a shallow bowl with caster sugar for dusting the doughnuts as they come out of the fryer.

When the oil is at the right temperature, fry the doughnuts in batches of 2 at a time until golden brown – don't try to cook any more or you'll reduce the temperature. They'll bob on the surface, so you need push them down lightly and flip them over halfway through. They'll take 2–3 minutes a side. If you find them difficult to move and handle, cut around the baking parchment they are sitting on and slide them onto a spatula; pop them in the oil, and the paper will detach immediately and can be removed with a pair of tongs.

When they're ready, remove them from the oil with a slotted spoon and toss them in the sugar before leaving to cool. They are best eaten on the same day, preferably while still warm. If you fancy filling them, leave to cool completely before trying one of the following ideas for fillings and dips:

HOW TO FILL

You'll need a piping bag if you want to fill your doughnuts; you can even buy longer, purpose-made piping nozzles to get right to their heart. Make a hole in the side of the doughnut and pipe in filling until you feel it start to swell and plump up. You can be more generous than the supermarkets ever are...

Recipe continues overleaf

JAM

The classic. Strawberry or raspberry are traditional, but whatever your most coveted conserve happens to be at the time will work. It is worth blending the jam to remove any large pieces of fruit, or it risks not making it through the piping nozzle. A total of 200–300g should do the lot.

RHUBARB AND CUSTARD

A marriage made in heaven and not out of bounds for vegans. It turns out that Bird's custard is vegan! Just use oat milk to make it up instead of regular milk. Make a 150ml batch, using a bit more powder than the packet suggests for a thicker set. Leave it to cool.

Cook 200g chopped rhubarb with 60g sugar and a tablespoon water for 10 minutes, until the rhubarb collapses. You want it to be nice and sharp to contrast with the creamy custard. Cool and blitz until smooth.

Pipe a shot of rhubarb purée into each doughnut, followed by a generous plug of custard.

APPLE, MAPLE AND CINNAMON

Add a good pinch of ground cinnamon to the caster sugar used for dusting the doughnuts as they come out of the oil. Peel, core and chop 2 large cooking apples and put them in a saucepan with 3 tablespoons maple syrup. Gently cook them down into a soft mush, then blend into a purée. Pipe a generous filling into each cinnamon-dusted doughnut.

CHOCOLATE DIPPERS

For something more snackable and shareable, shape your dough into smaller 20g balls. (They'll cook slightly quicker in the deep-fryer.) Add a good pinch each of ground cinnamon and nutmeg to the caster sugar used for dusting the doughnuts as they come out of the oil. Serve them warm, stacked alongside a bowl of warm Chocolate and Olive Oil Sauce (*see* page 154). Dip them into the chocolate sauce as you eat.

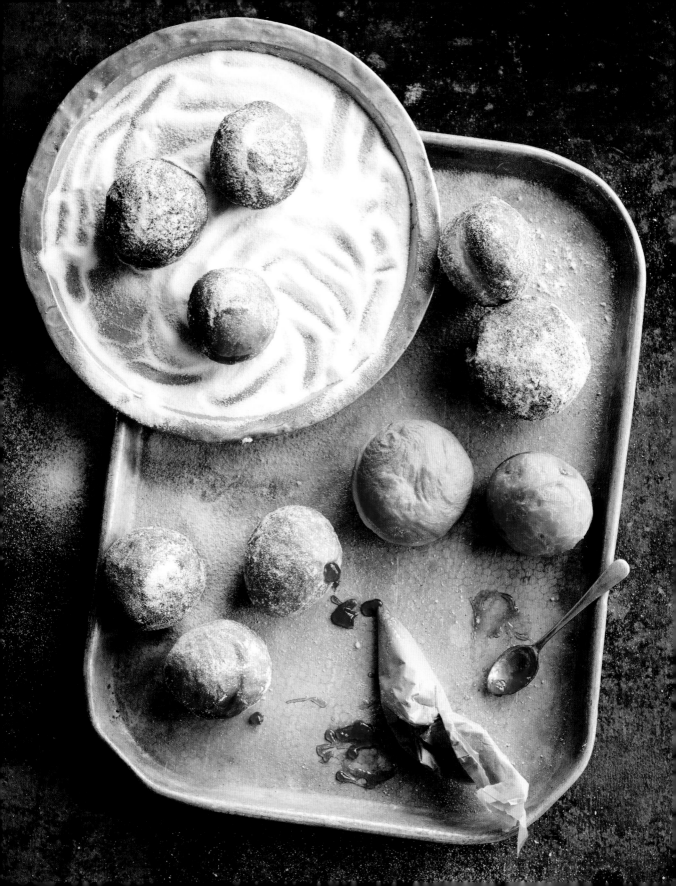

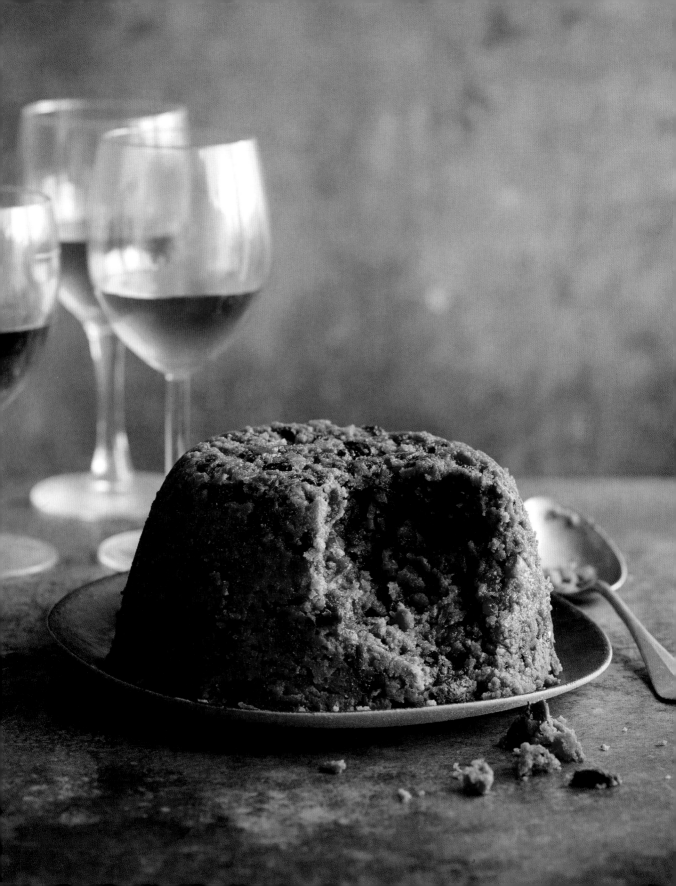

PRITCH'S CHRISTMAS PUD

SERVES 8

100ml dark stout
100ml brandy
150g sultanas
100g prunes, chopped
100g dried figs, chopped
50g dried cranberries
50g dried apricots, chopped
50g candied peel
150g vegan suet
150g light muscovado sugar
100g ground almonds
120g self-raising flour
finely grated zest
    and juice of 1 orange
1 large quince or
    cooking apple, grated
1 teaspoon mixed spice
1 whole blanched almond
a little flavourless vegetable oil

This is a mongrel of a recipe, tweaked over the years by new ideas, missing items, gathered suggestions and a need to use up what was in the cupboard. The large mix of dried fruits could be simplified, as long as it all adds up to the same weight. The sultanas and the candied peel are a must, though. I've got a bit of a free hand with the booze and tend to soak the fruit for a couple of weeks, and feed the odd bit of sherry and port in there too, just to really plump things up, so consider the 200ml suggested here just as a starting point! This is best made a few months before Christmas and stored somewhere cool, as the flavours mature over time. Some people suggest making it a whole year ahead, so that each Christmas you create and store the pudding for the following year. This recipe will fill a 1.5-litre pudding basin, enough to feed 8 people easily, or it can be split between 2 basins for smaller puds. Use the single almond in place of the traditional lucky silver penny. It saves the threat of choke hazards and/or dental costs. Whoever finds it is excused from the festive washing up.

Mix the booze with the dried and candied fruits and leave for at least 3 days, turning twice a day.

In a large bowl, mix all the other ingredients together except the whole blanched almond and the oil, then stir in the booze-soaked fruit.

Recipe continues overleaf

Grease a 1.5-litre pudding basin (or 2 smaller basins) with a little plain oil. Pack the mixture in and level it with the back of a spoon. Push the whole almond in at a random point. Top with a pleated circle of greaseproof paper, then a pleated sheet of foil. The pleats allow the pudding to expand without pushing the coverings off. Tie them on tightly with string. If your pudding basin has a lid, pop it on over the foil.

Place in a steamer basket and cook for 4 hours, topping up the water as needed.

Allow the pudding to cool completely. Remove the foil and paper, then wrap tightly in clingfilm and top with a fresh sheet of foil and the lid, if there is one. Store in a dark cool place until needed.

To reheat, remove the clingfilm and replace with greaseproof and foil, as before. Steam for 3 hours, until heated through. You can reheat it in a microwave, without the foil on, in 6–8 minutes – although, for some reason, this doesn't feel quite right.

RASPBERRY FRIANDS

MAKES 8

120g deodorized coconut oil,
    plus extra for greasing
100g self-raising flour, sifted
120g ground almonds
finely grated zest of ½ orange
pinch of salt
160g icing sugar, sifted,
    plus extra for dusting
100ml aquafaba (the liquid
    from a can of chickpeas)
120g raspberries

These almond cakes are a little more refined than a standard cupcake. They traditionally rely on whipped egg whites to add the rise, but we can employ the magic whiskable qualities of aquafaba that make vegan meringues possible. Although you can buy specific oval moulds for friands, this mixture needs baking in paper cases as it tends to stick in the tins, so a traditional cupcake shape is easier.

Preheat the oven to 170°C/Gas Mark 3. Line a 12 hole cupcake/small muffin tin with 8 paper cases. Melt the coconut oil in a pan until liquid. Leave to one side to cool slightly: you want it liquid but not too hot.

Mix the flour, almonds, orange zest and salt together in a bowl with one third of the icing sugar.

Tip the aquafaba into a clean bowl and whisk until light, foamy and doubled in size. This is easier with an electric mixer. Continue to whisk and add the rest of the icing sugar, bit by bit until glossy and meringue-like.

Tip the warm coconut oil into the flour and mix it together. Add one third of the aquafaba meringue and gently fold it in to loosen the mixture. Add the rest and fold it in gently but firmly until everything is just incorporated (too much mixing can knock the air out). Spoon the mixture into the cases; they should be about two-thirds full. Drop 2 or 3 raspberries into each one and transfer to the oven. Bake for 12–15 minutes, or until firm, risen and golden.

Allow to cool in the tins, then turn them out to cool on a wire rack. Dust lightly with a little icing sugar. Scoff.

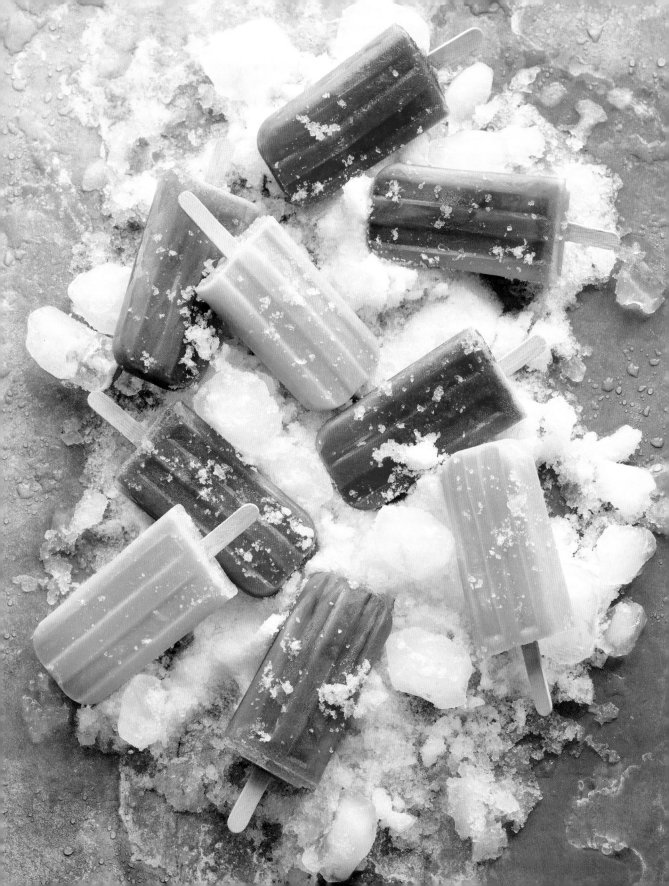

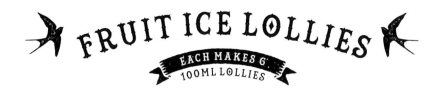

FRUIT ICE LOLLIES

EACH MAKES 6 100ML LOLLIES

The sweetness and yield of any lolly recipe will depend on the ripeness of the fruit, so you might have to tweak each mixture with more sugar and / or top it up with a little water. Sweetness is dulled by freezing, so make the mixtures slightly sweeter than you would usually.

You want the lollies to have some body to them, like good-quality smoothies, so press as many solids through the sieve as possible; you only want to remove any fibrous bits or seeds. Each recipe gives you the option to add a tot of booze to make the lollies a little more grown up, but the alcohol will increase the freezing time by a few hours. Either way, the trick to turning the lollies out is to dip the moulds in a jug of hot water for a few seconds to loosen them.

For each recipe, you'll need 6 x 100ml moulds and 6 x lolly sticks.

PREP: 10 MINUTES ★ FREEZE: 4–6 HOURS

PINEAPPLE, MANGO, and COCONUT

★

400g fresh pineapple, chopped
300g ripe mango, chopped
200g coconut milk, plus extra if needed
30g sugar, or to taste
1 tablespoon lime juice, or to taste (the amount will depend on the sweetness or sharpness of the fruit)
50ml white rum or Malibu (optional)

If you are feeling a little adventurous, mix 3 teaspoons salt with 2 teaspoons sugar and 1 teaspoon chilli powder and dab your lolly in this between bites. It is an acquired taste, but salt and chilli are common partners with pineapple and mango in India, South East Asia and Mexico.

Blitz everything together in a blender and pass it through a fine sieve into a large measuring jug, pushing through as many of the solids as possible. Add more coconut milk to make the total volume up to 600ml, if needed.

Taste and tweak the sweetness and sharpness with more sugar and lime juice, as needed. Pour into the moulds, add the lolly sticks and freeze.

KIWI, CUCUMBER and LIME
★

1 cucumber, chopped
4 kiwifruits, peeled
    and chopped
4 mint leaves
2 tablespoons lime juice,
    or to taste
30g sugar, or to taste
50ml gin (optional)

The kiwi is sharp, while the cucumber and mint are both mild and cooling.

Blitz everything together in a blender and press it through a fine sieve into a large measuring jug, pushing through as many of the solids as possible. Add water to make the total volume up to 600ml, if needed.

Taste and tweak the sweetness and sharpness with more sugar and lime juice, as needed. Pour into the moulds, add the lolly sticks and freeze.

STRAWBERRY, WATERMELON and BASIL,
★

300g strawberries
400g chopped
    watermelon flesh,
    large seeds removed
10–12 basil leaves
30g caster sugar, or to taste
2 tablespoons lemon juice,
    or to taste
50ml Pimms (optional)

Basil in an ice lolly sounds a bit odd, but its light, summery aniseed notes work really well with strawberries and watermelon.

Blitz everything together in a blender and press it through a fine sieve into a large measuring jug, pushing through as many of the solids as possible. Add water to make the total volume up to 600ml, if needed.

Taste and tweak the sweetness and sharpness with more sugar and lemon juice, as needed. Pour into the moulds, add the lolly sticks and freeze.

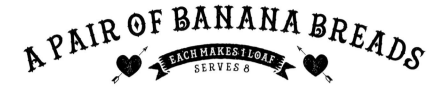

A PAIR OF BANANA BREADS

EACH MAKES 1 LOAF
SERVES 8

The perfect way to use up those over-ripe bananas that are turning black in the bowl, as their mushy texture and sickly-sweet taste are an ideal base for a cake. Here are two riffs on the same tune.

PREP: 10 MINUTES ★ COOK: 50 MINUTES

FRUIT and NUT

250g wholemeal
   self-raising flour
1 teaspoon baking powder
3 large over-ripe bananas
120g soft light brown sugar
60ml flavourless
   vegetable oil
60ml unsweetened
   almond milk
pinch of fine sea salt
½ teaspoon ground
   cinnamon
40g walnuts, chopped
30g sultanas, chopped

You can use hazelnuts, cashew nuts or even pine nuts instead of walnuts, if you prefer. Change up the dried fruit too: use cranberries, figs or prunes in the winter or dried pineapple, mango or apricots for a more exotic, summery feel.

Preheat the oven to 180°C (Gas Mark 4). Line a loaf tin (about 21 x 9cm) with baking parchment. Sift the flour and baking powder into a large mixing bowl.

Peel the bananas and mash them roughly with a fork in another bowl. Add the sugar, oil, milk, salt and cinnamon and whisk everything together. Tip the banana mixture into the bowl of flour, along with the walnuts and sultanas. Fold everything together until there is no dry flour visible. It needs to just come together into a batter; if you overmix it, the banana bread will be heavier.

Spoon the batter into the prepared tin and level it with the back of a spoon. I find the top tends to burn a little before the middle is set, so I cover the tin loosely with foil. Bake for 40 minutes, then remove the foil and bake for a further 10 minutes, or until a skewer comes out clean.

Cool for 15 minutes in the tin, then transfer to a wire rack to cool. It will last for a few days, if wrapped well.

CHOCOLATE and OLIVE OIL
★

250g wholemeal
   self-raising flour
3 tablespoons cocoa powder
1 teaspoon baking powder
3 large over-ripe bananas
120g soft light brown sugar
60g olive oil
60ml unsweetened
   almond milk
pinch of fine sea salt
70g vegan dark chocolate,
   roughly chopped

Not many people are aware of this, but Roald Dahl wrote a cookbook just before he died, in which he revealed his love of mashed banana with olive oil. I'm not sure it works as a snack, but folding them into a cake with some chocolate is scrumdiddlyumptious!

Follow the same instructions, but sift the cocoa powder with the flour and baking powder, then fold in the chopped chocolate instead of the walnuts and sultanas.

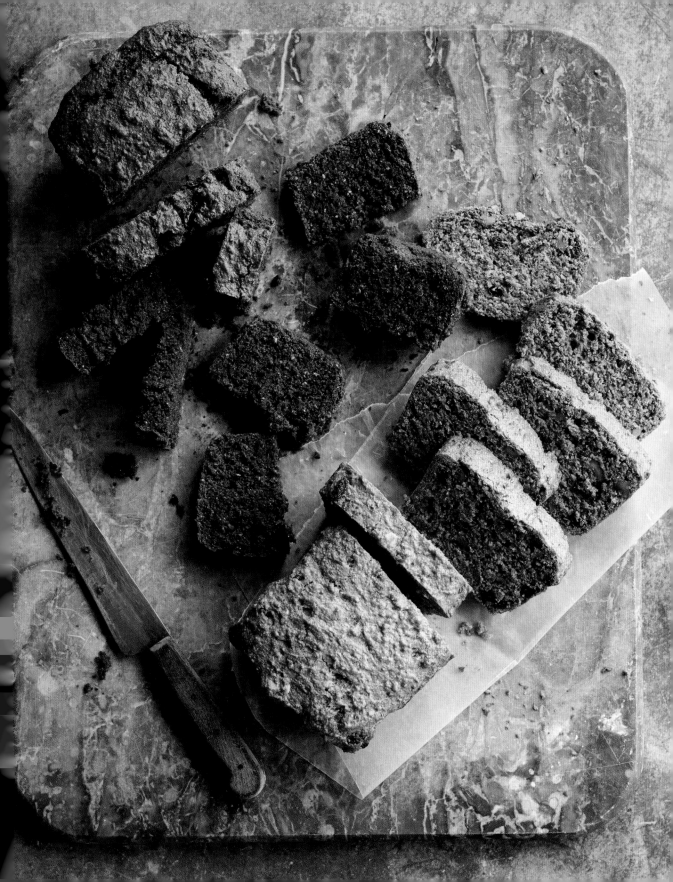

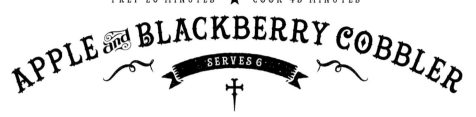

APPLE and BLACKBERRY COBBLER

SERVES 6

For the filling
800g apples, peeled,
    cored and chopped
200g blackberries
50g soft light brown sugar,
    or more to taste
½ teaspoon ground cinnamon
seeds from ½ vanilla pod

For the topping
150g deodorized coconut
    oil, fridge-cold and
    roughly chopped
300g plain flour
150g unrefined caster sugar
1 tablespoon baking powder
125ml unsweetened oat
    or almond milk

Cobbler is the new crumble, apparently. The topping is a clumsy scone mixture that rises during the bake. Leave nice gaps between the spoonfuls, so that the fruit can seep out in between the 'cobbles'. We are using coconut oil here instead of the traditional butter, to rub into the flour. This is easier if the oil is solid, so pop it in the fridge for 30 minutes before using if it feels a little soft at room temperature. The sharpness of the fruit is up to you, though it is often part of the charm of this pudding, especially if you use traditional cooking apples.

Mix the fruit in a saucepan with the sugar, cinnamon and vanilla seeds. Cook the fruit over a gentle heat for 5 minutes, until it has just begun to soften. Remove from the heat and transfer to a baking dish.

Preheat the oven to 180°C (Gas Mark 4).

Place the coconut oil in a large mixing bowl with the flour. Rub it together with your fingertips until it resembles coarse breadcrumbs. Mix in the sugar and baking powder.

Tip the milk into the flour mixture. Gently fold it together until just mixed – take care to not overmix.

Dollop and dot the mixture on top of the fruit in large spoonfuls, these are the 'cobbles'. It is fine (in fact, it is better) to have a few gaps in between them.

Bake for 30–40 minutes, or until the cobbles are cooked through and golden on top.

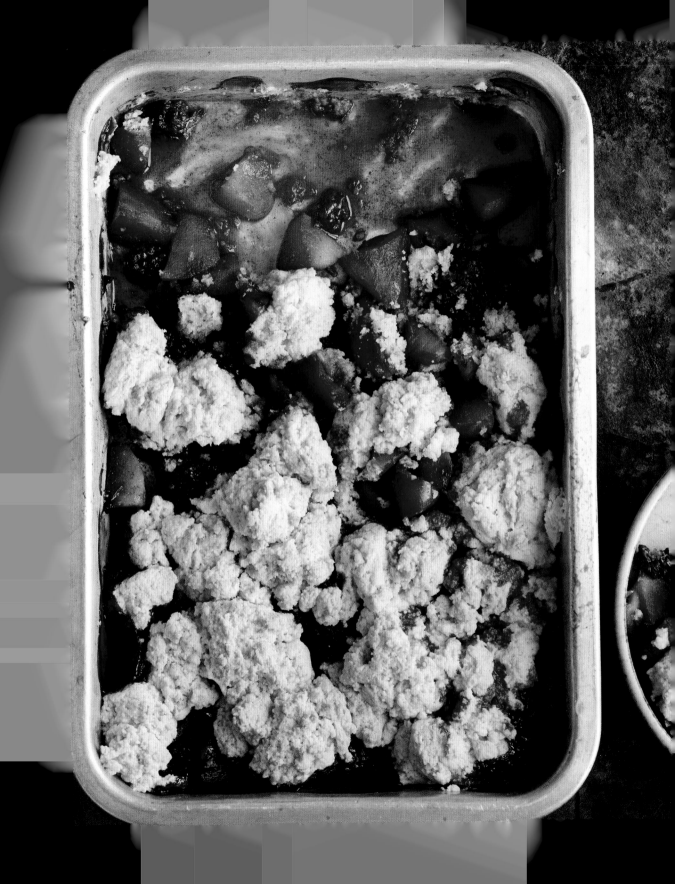

TURKISH DELIGHT BARBECUE PEACHES

SERVES 4

1 unwaxed lemon
100g unrefined caster sugar
70ml water
1 bay leaf
2 teaspoons rosewater,
    or to taste
4 peaches, halved and stoned
flavourless vegetable
    or sunflower oil
80g pistachio nuts,
    roughly chopped

This dish is about as delicate as I get, an antidote to too much stodge, pastry and chocolate. A proper summery recipe! Rosewater is a powerful thing. You just want a floral whiff; use too much and you'll feel like you are munching on potpourri. Feel free to switch the griddled peaches to nectarines, or even persimmons if you are feeling really fancy.

Use a peeler to pull 2 thin strips of zest from the lemon. Place them in a small saucepan with the sugar and the measured water. Add 2 tablespoons of lemon juice, then scrunch up the bay leaf and throw that in too. Slowly bring to the boil, stirring constantly to dissolve the sugar. Simmer for 1 minute, then turn off the heat and leave to cool. When it has cooled, add the rosewater: start with 1 teaspoon and taste, then add the rest to your taste a tiny bit at a time. I always keep this in the fridge, as I like the contrast of the cold syrup and the warm peaches. It keeps for weeks.

Heat a griddle pan or barbecue. Lightly brush the peaches with some oil (avoid strong-flavoured oils such as coconut or olive). Griddle them, cut-side down, over a medium heat, until nicely marked. This should take about 4 minutes; resist the temptation to play with them too much or they'll tend to stick or tear. Flip them and cook for a further 4 minutes or so until softened, the skins will wrinkle and pull away from the flesh when they are ready.

Divide the warm peaches between 4 bowls. Top each with a few spoonfuls of the cold syrup – it is very sweet, so a little goes a long way. Top with a scattering of pistachios.

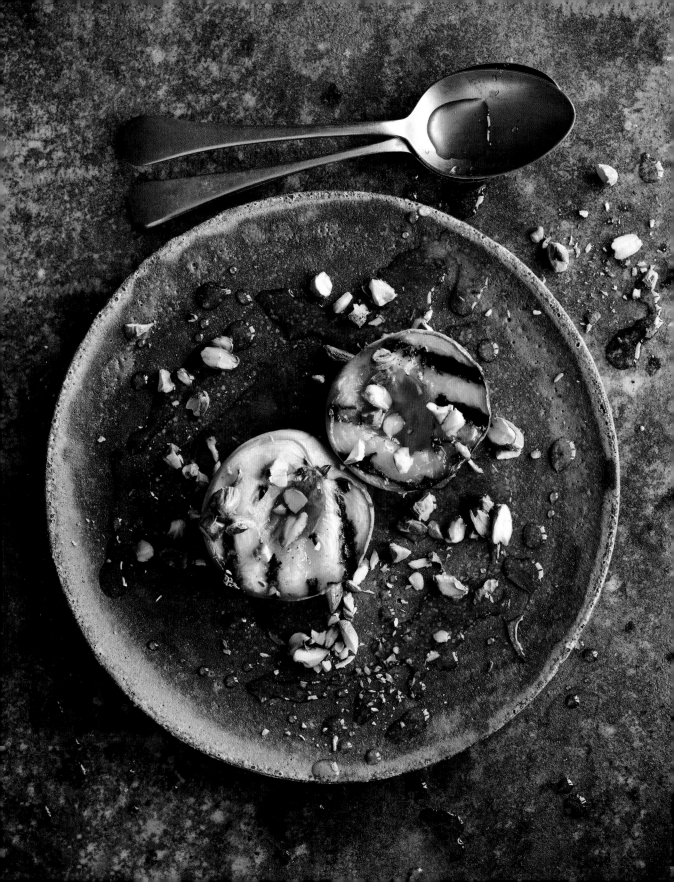

PUFFED PEARS WITH CHOCOLATE *and* OLIVE OIL SAUCE

SERVES 4

For the pears
4 firm pears
320g block of vegan
    puff pastry
unsweetened almond
    milk, to glaze
40g demerara sugar

For the basic poaching liquid
200g unrefined caster sugar
500ml water
juice of 1 unwaxed lemon,
    plus a strip of its zest
1 cinnamon stick
½ vanilla pod,
    seeds scraped out

**For the mulled wine
    poaching liquid**
150g unrefined caster sugar
500ml red wine
juice of 1 orange,
    plus a strip of its zest
1 cinnamon stick
3 cardamom pods, cracked
1 star anise
4 cloves
pinch of nutmeg

For the sauce
100g dark vegan
    cooking chocolate
4 tablespoons olive oil
4 tablespoons (60ml)
    boiling water
pinch of sea salt flakes

This is a bit of a showboater of a recipe. You'll need to poach the pears ahead of time and cool them before you attempt to wrap them in the pastry; warm pears would make the pastry impossible to handle. If you have perfectly ripe pears, though, you could make this recipe without poaching them first. I have included a mulled wine version of the poaching liquid in case you want to attempt that over the festive season, or just at any other time in midwinter. You could even reduce the mulled wine poaching liquid down until it's syrupy and serve it instead of the chocolate sauce, if you prefer. And on that subject, in theory, this chocolate sauce shouldn't work. It does everything you are told not to do with chocolate – such as adding water and heating it in a pan – but the olive oil seems to keep it all in check. With a bit of care and patience, it will come together. It wants to set as it cools, so serve it warm.

Peel the pears, leaving the stalks attached. Choose whether you are making the basic poaching liquid or the mulled wine version. Either way, place all the poaching ingredients together in a saucepan and bring to the boil over a medium heat, stirring to dissolve the sugar, then reduce the heat to a simmer. Add the pears to the pan and simmer very gently for 10 minutes, or until just soft to the tip of a knife. Turn the heat off and let the pears cool in the liquid. Store in the liquid until needed.

When you are ready to cook, preheat the oven to 180°C (Gas Mark 4). Roll the pastry out into a long, thin rectangle about 5mm thick. Cut it into 1.5cm-wide strips. Cut the very bottom of each pear away, so they can sit up straight. Starting from the bottom, wrap each pear in a tightly spiralled strip of pastry. You may need to join 2 or more strips together to complete each pear, but this is easily done by dabbing the ends of both with a little almond milk.

Once all the pears are wrapped, brush them lightly with almond milk and scatter over the demerara for crunch. Transfer them to a baking tray and cook in the oven for 20 minutes, or until golden.

When ready, leave them to rest for 10 minutes, which gives you just enough time to make the sauce.

Break the chocolate into small pieces and place them in a small saucepan. Add the olive oil and water. Now, swirl and roll the pan so that the hot water starts to melt the chocolate, but resist the temptation to mix or whisk it. It might need a little more heat to keep it going, so place the pan over a low heat to give it a nudge. Don't keep it on the heat for too long and don't let it get anywhere near boiling. When the chocolate seems to have almost lost it shape, you can use a use a metal spoon to stir it together. It should come together into a smooth glossy sauce. Add the pinch of salt and serve immediately, spooning a pool of sauce on to each warm plate and sitting a pastry-wrapped pear on top.

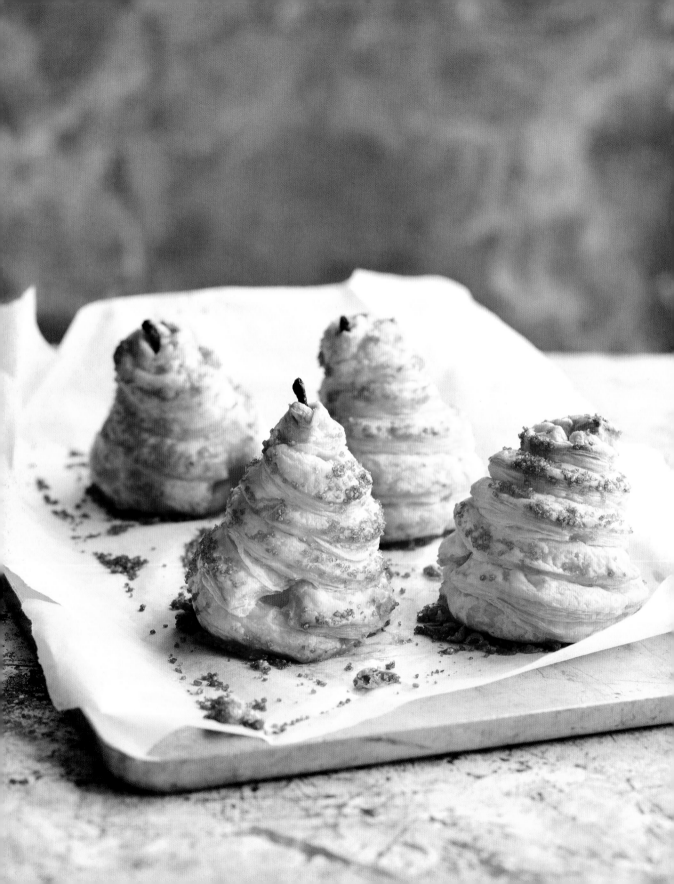

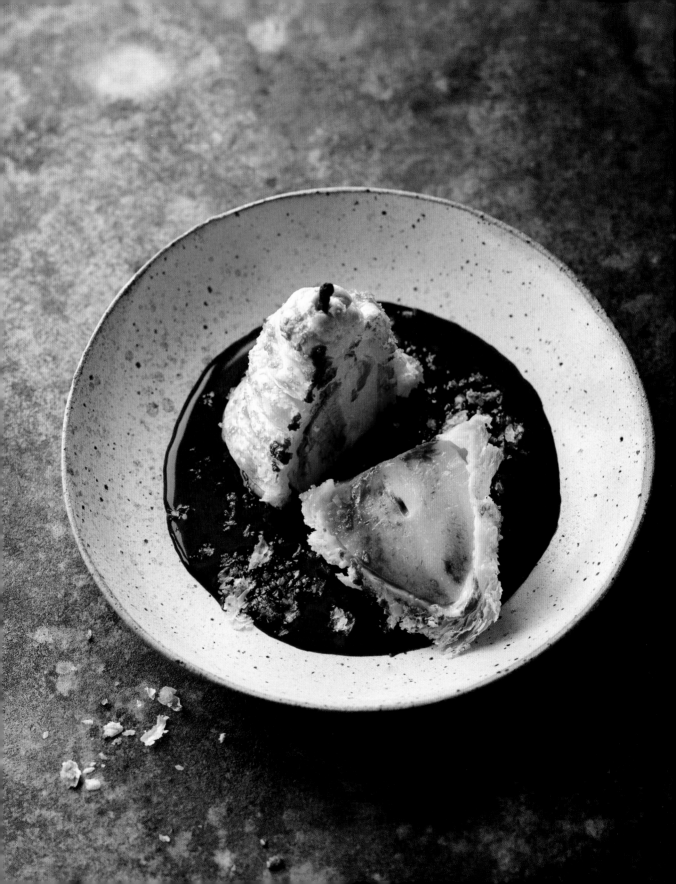

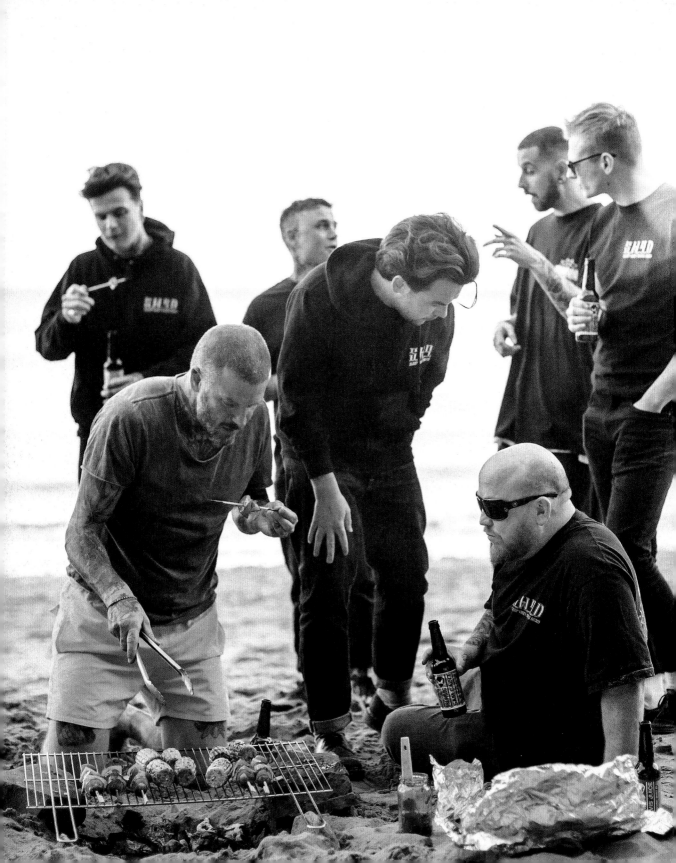

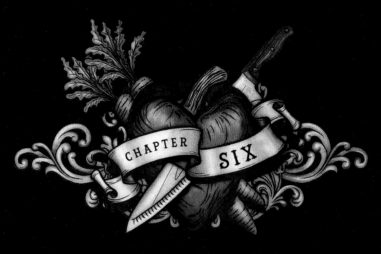

DINNER
WITH
MATES

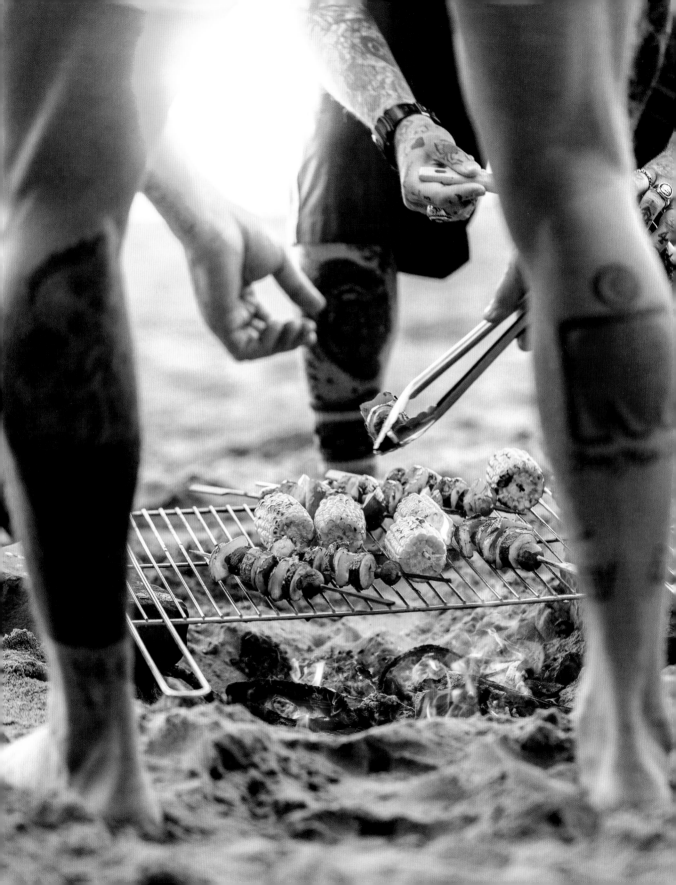

Good things can happen when you share food. You don't even need an excuse like a birthday bash, just pin down a date and get everyone together round a table. I know we all say we're so busy these days... and it's true. We're either glued to screens or chasing work rather than just being together and enjoying the simple stuff, such as a proper catch-up. A bit of grub. A beer and a laugh. I reckon it does more for your mental health than any supplement!

The dinners in this chapter are made for sharing. If you are too busy to cook them all, then take the pressure off and get everyone to bring one of the dishes each, and see if you can convert any of your non-plant-based friends to vegan grub. They'll want to, after this lot! Better still, get a couple of friends over early and make cooking the dinner part of the get-together. You'll be surprised where you can take the conversation when eyes are focussed on chopping veg. If you are worried about a friend, get them round and make a curry together. We all need a bit of a hand sometimes. Food isn't the answer, but it really can help.

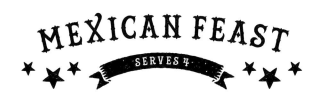

MEXICAN FEAST

SERVES 4

This is a proper get-in-there meal that is full of colour and flavour, and great for sharing. Get your mates round to help prep everything too. More fun than just catching up in the pub.

PREP: 15 MINUTES, PLUS 20 MINUTES MACERATING

CHOPPED SALSA

★

½ red onion,
    finely chopped
1 garlic clove,
    finely chopped
½ cucumber, deseeded
    and finely chopped
300g tomatillos
    or tomatoes,
    roughly chopped
1 red chilli, deseeded
    and finely chopped
3 tablespoons olive oil
salt
juice of 1 lime
leaves from a small
    bunch of coriander,
    finely chopped
leaves from a small
    bunch of mint,
    finely chopped

Tomatillos are a relative of the tomato, sharper and sourer, and with a papery husk that needs removing before using. You might be able to get some in the middle of summer but don't fret if not, you can just use some regular toms instead. Add the herbs just before using, as the acidity of tomatillos or tomatoes can knock the freshness out of them if left for too long.

Place the onion, garlic, cucumber, tomatillos or tomatoes and chilli in a mixing bowl with the olive oil. Mix together and season with salt and lime juice to your taste; though I say, go for it! (You'll find you need less lime if using the tomatillos.)

Leave the salsa to macerate (mingle and develop flavours) for at least 20 minutes.

When ready to serve, fold in the freshly chopped herbs and tweak the seasoning, if it needs it.

CHILLI NON CARNE TEMPEH TOSTADAS

★

2 tablespoons olive oil,
  plus extra for brushing
1 large onion,
  finely chopped
1 red pepper, deseeded
  and finely chopped
400g tempeh
2 garlic cloves,
  finely chopped
½ tablespoon ground cumin
1 teaspoon ground
  coriander
½ teaspoon sweet
  smoked paprika
¼ teaspoon ground
  cinnamon
chilli flakes, to taste
1 teaspoon dried oregano
400g can chopped tomatoes
4 corn tortillas
1 Little Gem lettuce,
  shredded
1 avocado, peeled,
  pitted and sliced
vegan cheese or crème
  fraîche, to serve
  (optional)
salt and pepper

A tostada is a crispy tortilla that you can load with whatever filling floats your plant-based boat. I've chosen a classic chilli, using tempeh in place of minced meat. When fried, the tortillas crisp up like a giant nacho chip. Pressing them into a bowl as they cool gives them a rounded shape, so you can properly load and fill them!

Warm 2 tablespoons of olive oil in a saucepan over a gentle heat. Add the onion and pepper and cook until starting to soften.

Meanwhile, roughly chop or crumble the tempeh. Add it to the saucepan, increase the heat and fry for 5 minutes, until it has lightly coloured.

Throw in the garlic, spices and oregano and cook for 1 more minute, stirring to make sure the spices don't stick, then tip in the tomatoes. Half-fill the empty tomato tin with water and tip that in, too. Bring to the boil, then reduce the heat to a simmer, season with salt and pepper and cook gently for 20 minutes, until you have a thick, rich sauce. Taste and tweak the seasoning with more salt, pepper and chilli flakes to your liking.

Put a frying pan over a medium heat, while you find 4 shallow dessert bowls to shape the tortillas in.

One at a time, brush the tortillas on both sides with olive oil. Place in the frying pan and fry over a medium heat for about 1 minute on each side, until nicely coloured. Remove from the pan and immediately press into a bowl. Leave to cool; they'll crisp up and hold their shape. Repeat to fry and shape all 4 tortillas.

When cool, divide the shredded lettuce between the tortillas, followed by the warm tempeh chilli. Top with avocado and the vegan cheese or crème fraîche, if using.

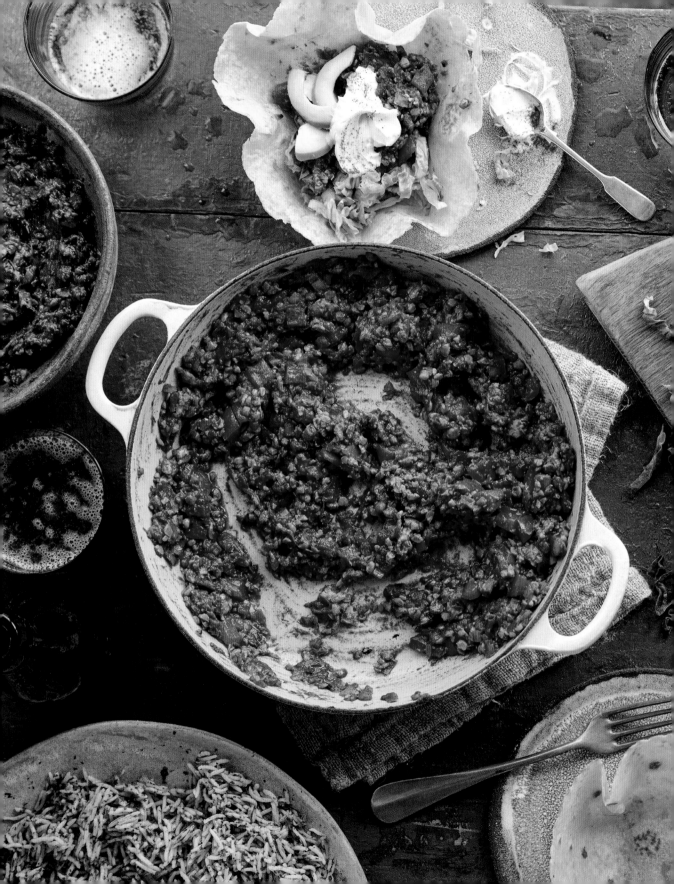

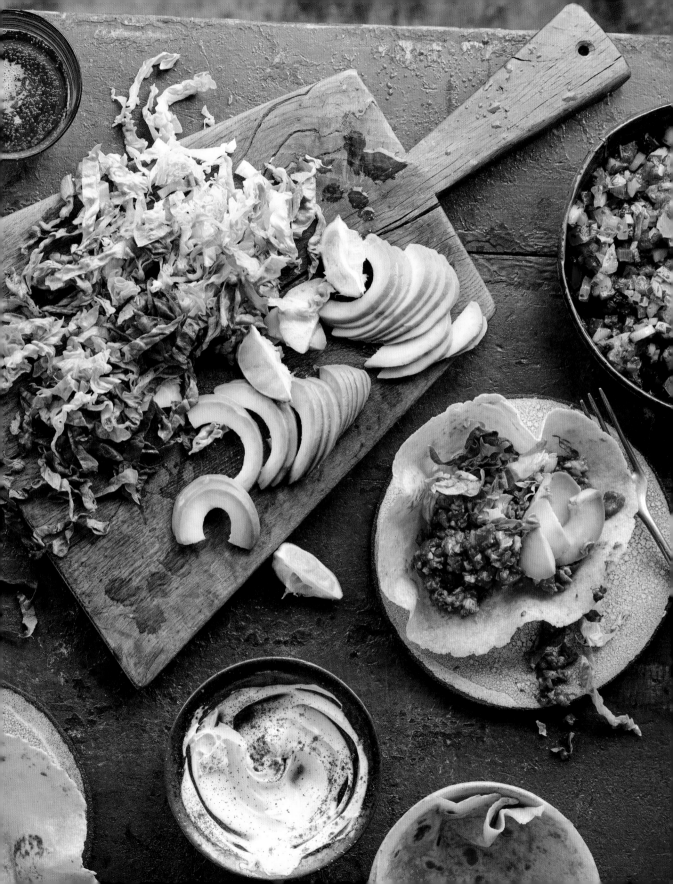

FRIJOLES

olive oil
1 red onion, finely chopped
2 x 400g cans black beans
2 garlic cloves,
    finely chopped
1 red chilli, finely chopped
1 teaspoon ground cumin
juice of 1 lime
salt

Also known as refried beans, these couldn't be easier to make. The seasoning is simple and straightforward, as they are almost always served alongside other more heavily seasoned dishes. They make a good dip, too.

Heat 2 tablespoons of oil in a saucepan over a gentle heat. Add the onion and cook for 10 minutes, until starting to soften.

Meanwhile, open and drain 1 tin of black beans. Open the other too, but retain the liquid.

Add the garlic, chilli and cumin to the pan and cook for 1 more minute before tipping in all the beans and the reserved liquid from the second can. Season with salt and cook over a low heat for 10 minutes, until the beans are nice and soft.

Blend or mash the beans. Taste and tweak with more salt, if needed, and a squeeze or 2 of lime juice for a bit of zing.

GREEN RICE

2 green peppers, or 4 fresh
   poblano peppers, if you
   can find them
olive oil
300g basmati or other
   long-grain rice, rinsed
bunch of coriander, any
   coarse stalks removed
80g baby spinach
1 garlic clove
1 green chilli, deseeded
   and chopped
salt

This is bursting with green goodness! Blitzing all the greens together separately means you can stir them in at the very end, keeping all the bright, fresh colour. The roasted peppers are traditional, but you can blend them from raw, if you want, to speed everything up.

Preheat your oven to 200°C (Gas Mark 6). Rub the peppers lightly with oil, place them in the oven and roast until blistered and blackened on the outside, 25–30 minutes. Remove from the oven, pop them in a bowl and cover with a plate; this makes the skins easier to remove later.

Cook the rice according to the packet instructions.

While the rice cooks, peel away and discard the skins and seeds from the peppers. Place the peppers in a blender with the coriander, spinach, garlic and chilli. Add a dash of water and blend into a thick, bright green paste.

When the rice is cooked, stir the greens in and tweak the seasoning with salt.

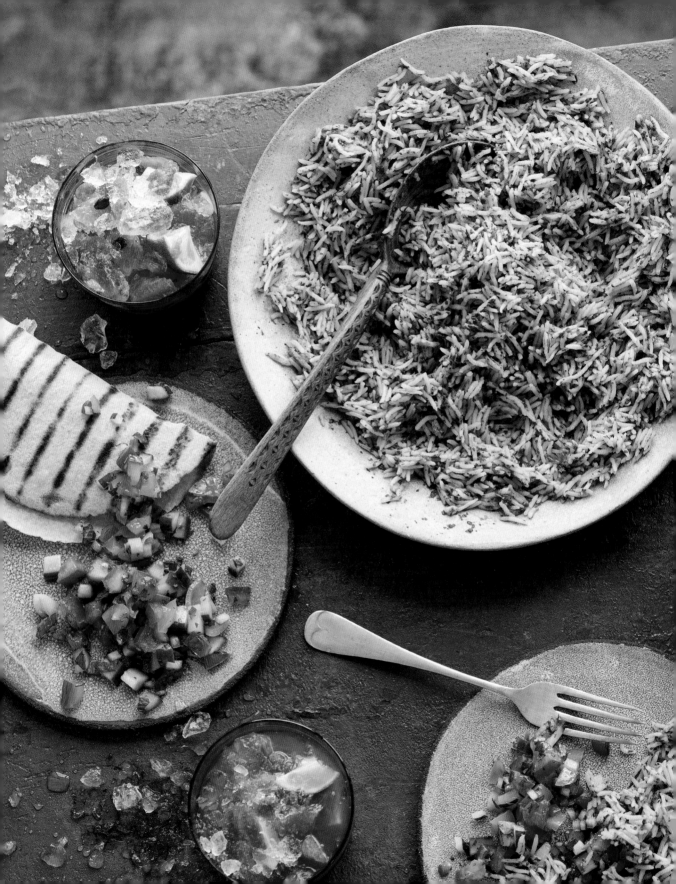

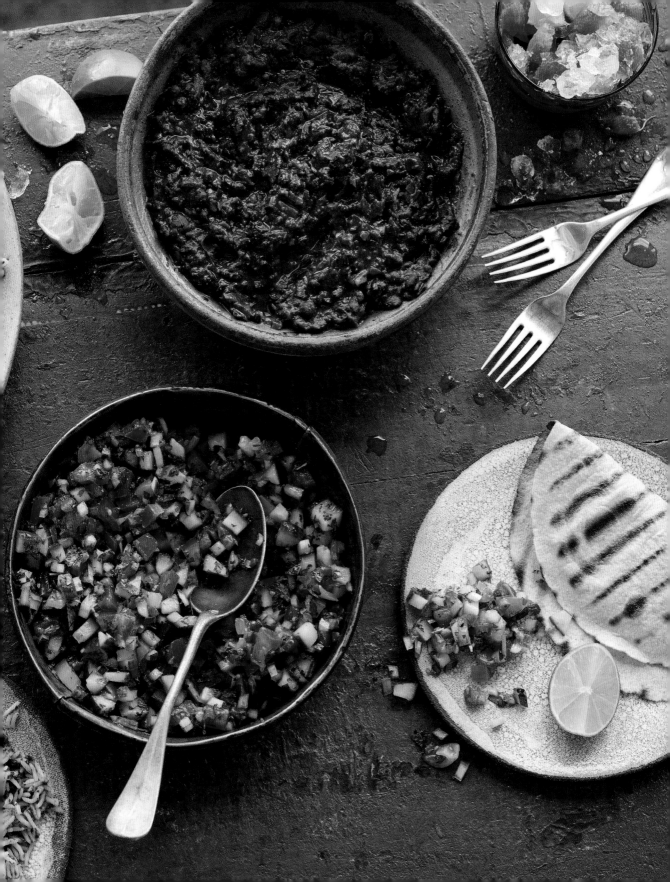

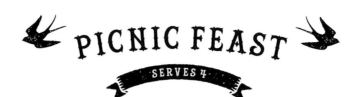

PICNIC FEAST

SERVES 4

Perfect for a properly hot day where you all want to get outside, get together, and have a laugh over a decent spread. Everything can be made in advance, then chilled and transported.

PREP: 10 MINUTES, PLUS 1 HOUR CHILLING

GAZPACHO

1 thick slice of stale
   sourdough bread
800g very ripe tomatoes,
   roughly chopped
1 red pepper, deseeded
   and roughly chopped
½ cucumber, peeled and
   roughly chopped
2 garlic cloves, chopped
4 tablespoons olive oil,
   plus extra to serve
salt
2 tablespoons sherry
   vinegar or red wine
   vinegar, or to taste

The idea of a cold soup doesn't always appeal... where does that end and a vegetable smoothie begin?? This is one of the few that really works, ideally on a blisteringly hot day. It sounds a bit pretentious I know, but this is one dish where quality and seasonal ingredients are really important, as you can't hide behind any heat or strong seasoning. You need ripe veg and the kind of oil and vinegar that you wouldn't mind swigging straight from the bottle. If you want to take this on a picnic, transport it in a Thermos flask. It will stay fridge-cold for a few hours.

Remove the crust from the bread and tear it into small pieces. Place them in a blender along with the tomatoes, pepper, cucumber, garlic and oil. Blend until smooth. Add a little cold water to thin the gazpacho, if it seems too thick.

Taste and season with salt and vinegar to your liking; the amount you need will depend on the acidity of the tomatoes.

Pass the gazpacho through a fine sieve to remove any lumps, pushing through as much as you can with the back of a spoon. Place it in the fridge to chill for at least an hour.

Serve in chilled bowls, if possible, and finish with a drizzle of olive oil.

ASPARAGUS 'CHEESE' STRAWS
★

plain flour, for dusting
200g block of vegan
    puff pastry
1 tablespoon Dijon mustard
50g vegan cheese,
    grated (optional)
2 tablespoons
    nutritional yeast
½ tablespoon chopped
    rosemary leaves
chilli flakes, to taste
12 fat asparagus spears
olive oil, for brushing
salt and pepper

A surprising amount of puff pastry on the market is vegan now, so you should have no problem getting your hands on some. For this recipe, whatever seems the most Parmesan-like of the vegan cheeses you can find is best. If you would rather not use a cheese substitute, double the amount of nutritional yeast instead, to boost the savoury flavours.

Dust your work surface with a little flour. Roll the pasty out into a long rectangle, about 3mm thick. Spread the mustard thinly over the pastry, then sprinkle over the cheese (if using), yeast, rosemary and chilli flakes.

Fold the pastry in half and roll it back out into a rectangle. Cut it into 12 long strips and pop in the fridge to chilli for 20 minutes.

Meanwhile, preheat the oven to 200°C (Gas Mark 6).

Trim away any tough ends from the asparagus. Remove the pastry from the fridge. Coil each asparagus spear in a spiral of pastry and lay them on a baking tray. Brush the pastry lightly with olive oil and season with a pinch of salt and a grind of pepper.

Bake for 15–20 minutes, until the pastry is golden and the asparagus tender. Wolf down hot, or cool on a wire rack and pack for a picnic.

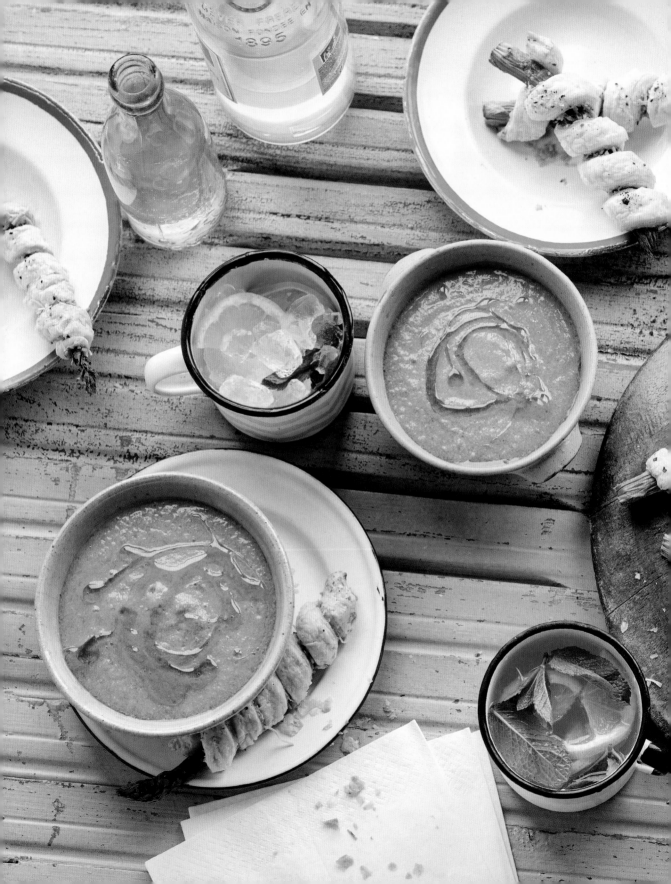

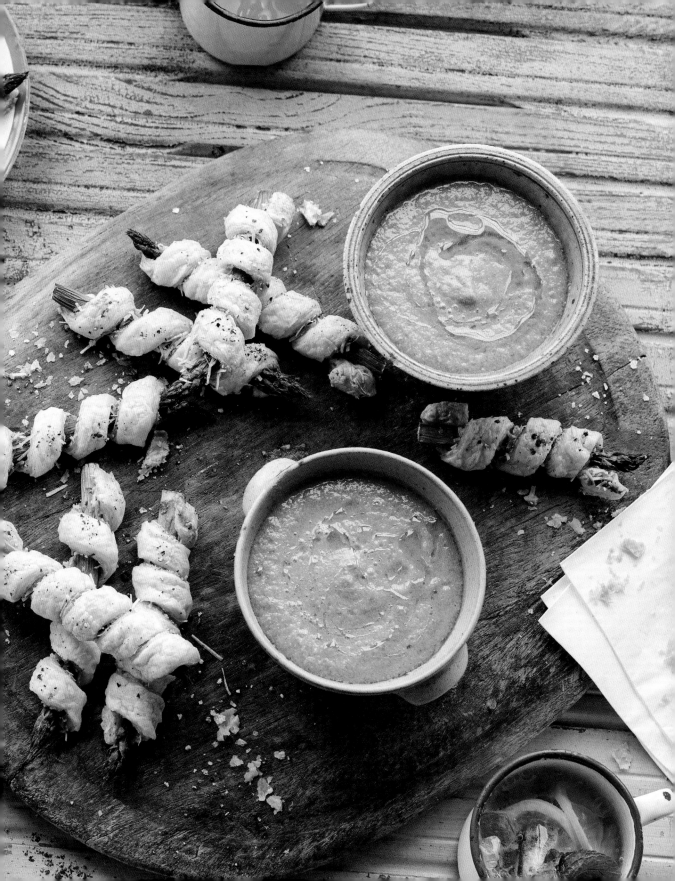

GREEN TABBOULEH

★

150g bulgur wheat
3 tablespoons olive oil
200g cherry tomatoes,
    quartered
1 courgette, coarsely grated
100g French beans,
    very thinly sliced
2 spring onions,
    thinly sliced
leaves from a large bunch
    of parsley, chopped
leaves from a small bunch
    of mint, chopped
juice of 1 lemon
salt and pepper

I prefer to leave all the veg raw in this and spend time thinly slicing them… think of it as a sort of therapy! You can keep everything in larger pieces and cook the courgette and beans first if you like, but if the season is right, everything should be fine. You can even make this the night before, but don't add the herbs until the day you want to eat it, or they can discolour.

Boil your kettle. Place the bulgur wheat in a heatproof bowl and mix in 1 tablespoon of olive oil and a pinch of salt. Tip in enough boiling water to cover by 1cm, stick a plate on top and leave it for 15 minutes, to plump up.

Use this time to prepare the veg and place them in a bowl with the remaining 2 tablespoons of oil and a good pinch of salt.

Fluff up the bulgur wheat with a fork and add it to the mixing bowl along with the herbs and a good squeeze of lemon juice. Mix well and tweak the seasoning with more salt, pepper and lemon juice to taste. Pack up and take on a picnic.

POTATO and ONION TORTILLA
★

3 tablespoons olive oil
1 large onion, sliced
500g waxy new potatoes
100g gram (chickpea) flour
250ml warm water
½ teaspoon black salt, or
  regular salt (black salt
  can be found online or
  in Indian supermarkets)
1 garlic clove,
  finely chopped
salt and pepper

Gram (chickpea) flour has the handy quality of setting as it cooks, acting as a perfect binder. Black salt adds an interesting sulphurous note that apes the traditional egg, but it isn't vital to the final dish, more of a nice-to-have-if-you-can.

Heat 2 tablespoons of olive oil in a 24cm nonstick frying pan. Add the onion and a pinch of salt. Cook over a gentle heat for 20 minutes, until soft and sweet.

Meanwhile, place the potatoes in a saucepan of cold salted water over a high heat. Bring to the boil and cook for 5 minutes, then drain. When cool enough to handle, slice them into thin discs. Add the potatoes to the onions along with another 1 tablespoon of oil. Cook over a medium heat for 8–10 minutes, until the potatoes soften. Turn them occasionally, but avoid breaking them up.

While the potatoes cook, make the batter by whisking the gram flour with the measured water, until any lumps have disappeared. Add the black salt or regular salt, garlic and some black pepper. Tip the batter into the frying pan. Prod and poke the mixture so that it runs evenly through it, then level the top out. Cook over a medium heat for 6–7 minutes, until set.

You now want to flip the tortilla so that you can get some colour on both sides. Place a plate on top of the pan and place a cloth on top to avoid burning your hands. Press down on the plate and, in one swift movement, flip the pan over so that tortilla turns out on to the plate. Place the pan back over the heat and slide the now inverted tortilla back in. Cook for a further 4–5 minutes, until the bottom is coloured too. If this all feels a bit perilous, you could slide the pan under a grill to brown the top, but you don't get the perfect flying saucer shape of a traditional tortilla.

Slide the tortilla out of the pan and leave to cool for at least 10 minutes before serving, or pack it up and take it on your picnic.

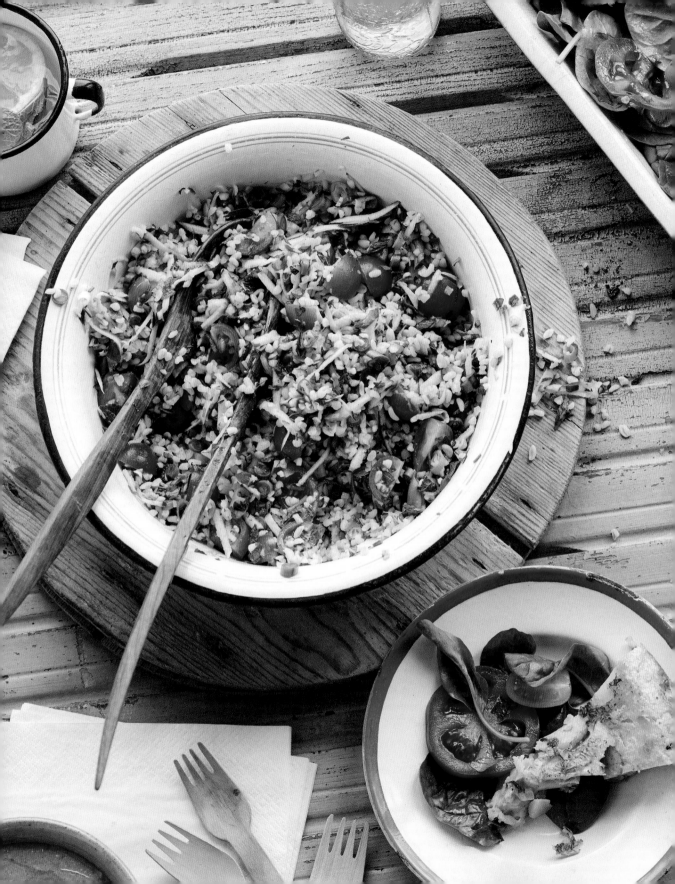

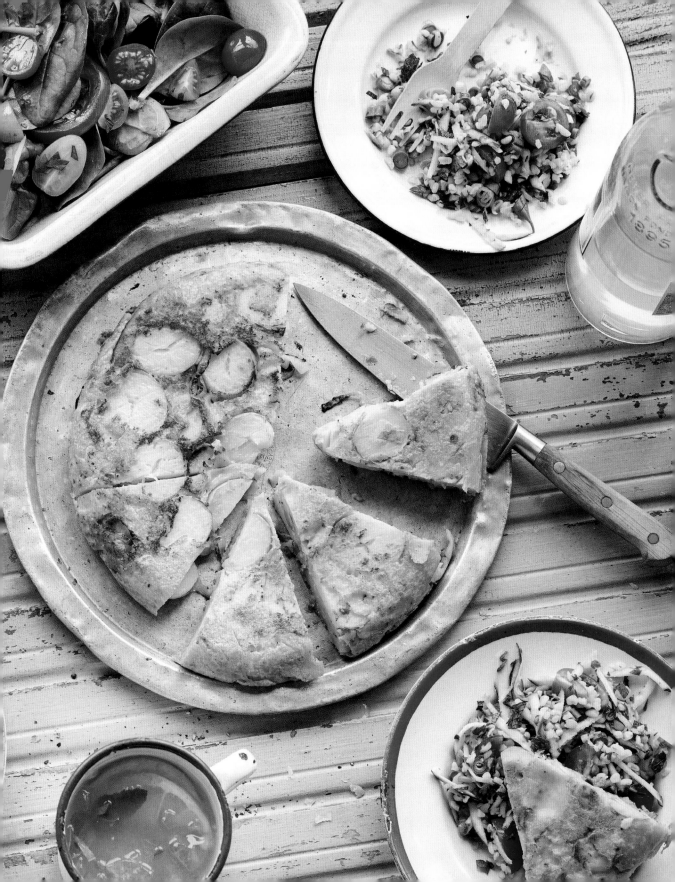

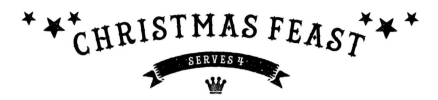

CHRISTMAS FEAST

SERVES 4

This is a proper vegan celebration, with loads of colour and flavour. No one will feel like they are missing out! Serve these dishes with loads of Gravy (see page 122). For dessert, there is no other option than Pritch's Christmas Pud (see page 141).

PREP: 10 MINUTES ★ COOK: 40–50 MINUTES

PARSNIPS and CARROTS WITH CLEMENTINES and SPICES

600g carrots, peeled
   and chopped into
   3cm angled pieces
400g parsnips, peeled
   and chopped into
   3cm angled pieces
1 cinnamon stick
1 star anise
3 cloves
1 bay leaf
2 clementines,
   sliced into discs
3 tablespoons light
   olive oil
dash of Marsala wine
   (optional)
salt and pepper

These sweet roots are baked with all the flavours of Christmas: a few traditional mulling spices and some zesty clementines. I cover them for the first half of cooking so that they lightly steam, which helps to cook them evenly, as winter roots can be a little tough.

Preheat the oven to 200°C (Gas Mark 6). Throw everything together in a large roasting tin, adding a dash of water if you're not using the Marsala. Season well with salt and pepper, cover tightly with foil and pop into the oven to roast for 20 minutes.

Remove the foil. Give everything a gentle stir and return to the oven for a further 20–30 minutes, until tender and starting to colour. Pluck out the spices and bay leaf and serve immediately.

BEETROOT WELLINGTON
★

3 large beetroots, scrubbed
10 black peppercorns
3 star anise
½ cinnamon stick
2 bay leaves
2 tablespoons flavourless
    vegetable oil (such as
    sunflower), plus extra
    for brushing
1 red onion, finely chopped
250g chestnut mushrooms,
    finely chopped
2 garlic cloves,
    finely chopped
½ teaspoon thyme leaves
150g Puy lentils
175ml red wine
250ml vegetable stock,
    preferably dark and
    with mushrooms
    (see page 121)
250g baby spinach
400g block of vegan
    puff pastry
salt and pepper

A plant-based take on a classic. When you cut the Wellington open, the different colours look amazing thanks to the beetroot.

Chuck the beetroots in a pan of cold water with the whole spices and bay leaves and a generous seasoning of salt. Bring to the boil, then reduce the heat to a simmer and cook for 40–60 minutes. You may need to top the water up as you go. Leave to cool.

Meanwhile, warm the oil in a saucepan and cook the onion and mushrooms for 5 minutes, until they begin to soften. Add the garlic, thyme, lentils and wine. Cook for 2–3 minutes to reduce the wine by half, then tip in the stock and bring to a simmer. Cook, uncovered, for 30 minutes or so, until the lentils are very soft and the liquid absorbed. You want to end up with a thick, spreadable mixture. Season and leave to cool.

While the lentils cook, put a kettle on to boil. Place the spinach in a deep bowl and cover with boiling water. Give it a stir for 1 minute, then drain and cool immediately under cold water. Drain again and squeeze out any excess water. Coarsely chop the leaves.

Preheat the oven to 200°C (Gas Mark 6). Drain the beetroots, slide their skins off and cut away the tops and bottoms. Cut each one in half from top to bottom, giving you 6 stout hemispheres.

Roll the pastry out between 2 sheets of baking parchment into a large rectangle, about 5mm thick. Fold the spinach into the lentils and spread it evenly over the pastry, leaving a 2cm gap along one long edge. Place the beetroot pieces evenly in a row down the centre, end to end. Brush the exposed edge of the pastry with a little water. Gently lift the pastry up and over to completely encase the beetroot, pressing the damp edge down to seal. Crimp the open ends together. Transfer to a baking sheet, brush with a little oil and lightly score the top. Transfer to the oven and bake for 20–25 minutes, until golden and cooked through.

POLENTA and ROSEMARY ROASTIES

★

1.2kg King Edward potatoes
3 garlic cloves
1 bay leaf
10g rosemary sprigs
4 tablespoons light olive oil
4 tablespoons polenta
salt and pepper

King Edwards are universally recognized as the top dog for perfect roasties, but any floury spud will work. A dusting of polenta is a great trick to give you good crispy edges: it draws out some of the surface moisture as well as giving a light, crunchy coating. For a perfectly seasoned spud, make sure you season the water you boil them in heavily. They'll draw up some of the salt as they cook, along with any other aromatics that are added to the water.

Peel the spuds and cut them into generous, equal-sized roasties. Place them into a large pan of cold, well-salted water. Give the garlic cloves a bash to split them open and throw them into the pan too, along with the bay leaf and half the rosemary.

Bring the water to the boil, then reduce the heat to a simmer and cook the spuds for about 12 minutes, until mostly cooked through. Drain them well and leave to steam in the colander for a few minutes. Discard the garlic, bay and rosemary from the pan.

Meanwhile, preheat the oven to 200°C (Gas Mark 6). Add the oil to a large roasting tin and pop it in the oven to heat up.

Dust the potatoes with the polenta, then give them a turn to coat and toss them to rough up the edges slightly.

Remove the tin from the oven, being careful of the hot oil. Add the potatoes, turn them gently to coat in the oil and season with salt and pepper. Transfer to the oven and roast for 20 minutes, then give them shake and a turn and roast for a final 20–30 minutes, until golden and crisp. While they roast, strip the leaves from the remaining rosemary and coarsely chop them.

When the potatoes are ready, mix the chopped rosemary into the tray. Leave for 5 minutes before serving; the residual heat of the roasting tin will infuse the potatoes with the scent of the rosemary.

SPROUTS, CABBAGE and CHESTNUTS WITH CRISPY GARLIC

★

8 large garlic cloves, peeled
300g Brussels sprouts,
    halved or quartered,
    depending on size
4 tablespoons deodorized
    coconut oil
120g cooked chestnuts,
    coarsely chopped
½ small Savoy cabbage,
    shredded
salt and pepper

Roasted sprouts are banging, but with everything else going on in this meal you won't have space in your oven for those, so get all Oriental and use a wok instead.

Put a pan of salted water on to the heat. Throw in the garlic cloves and bring to the boil, then reduce to a gentle simmer. Poach gently for 10 minutes until soft to a knife tip. Remove with a slotted spoon. Keep the water on the heat.

Add the sprouts to the pan of water and cook for 3 minutes, until almost cooked through. Drain.

When the garlic cloves are cool enough to handle, cut them into quarters.

Heat 2 tablespoons of the oil in a wok over a medium heat. Add the chestnuts and a pinch of salt and fry for 2 minutes. Add the garlic and cook for a few more minutes, until both the chestnuts and garlic are golden. Remove from the wok.

Wipe the wok clean, add 2 more tablespoons of oil and return to the heat. Add the cabbage and a pinch of salt. Stir-fry over a medium-high heat for 2 minutes, until starting to wilt, then throw in the part-cooked sprouts. Stir-fry for 2–3 more minutes, until everything is tender. Return the chestnuts and garlic, toss together for 30 seconds to warm them through, then adjust the seasoning to taste and serve immediately.

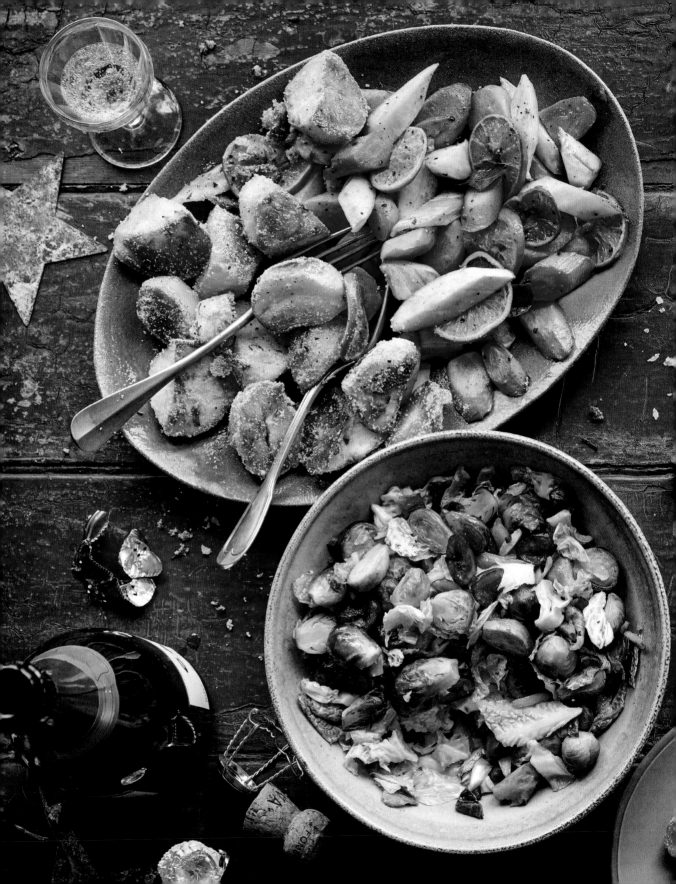

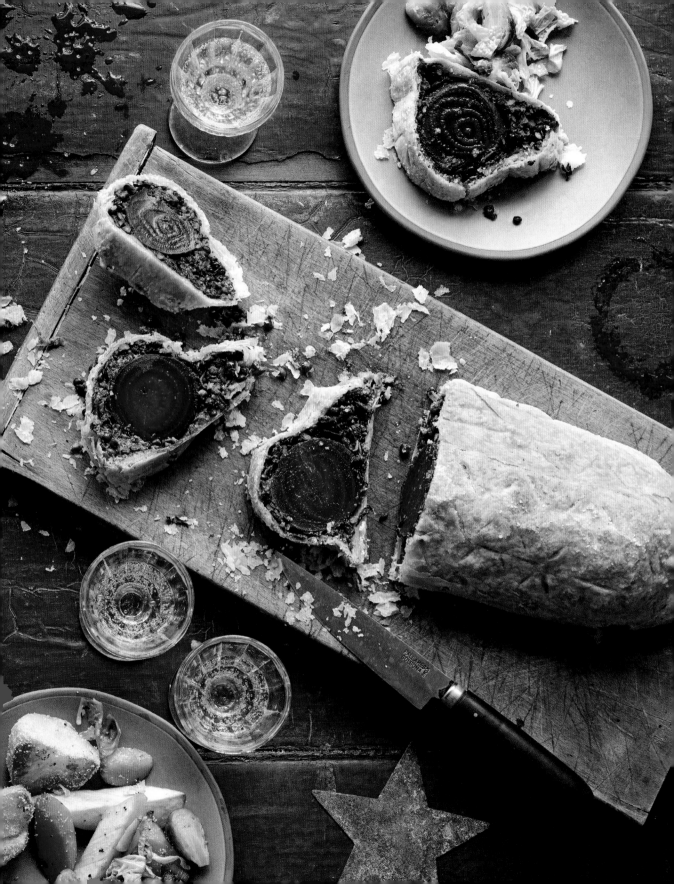

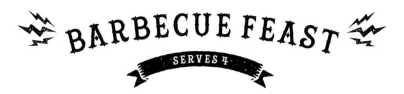

BARBECUE FEAST
SERVES 4

For perfect barbecuing, you need three distinct zones in your fire... I've learned this the hard way! First off, you need a deep area of hot glowing embers on one side for high-heat direct cooking. In the middle, rake a thinner layer of ebbing embers for cooler indirect cooking. At the other end, keep a fire-free space to hold cooked food, or as a 'time out' zone for food that needs to come off the heat for a while. These different areas allow you to cook different things at different speeds at the same time, while dodging the risk of a cremated dinner.

PREP: 10 MINUTES, PLUS 30 MINUTES MARINATING ★ COOK: 20 MINUTES

SPICY SMOKEY SQUASH
★

2 garlic cloves,
    finely chopped
2 teaspoons ground cumin
3 tablespoons
    chipotle paste
3 tablespoons olive oil
1 large butternut squash,
    cut into 8 wedges
    lengthways, soft seedy
    core scooped out from
    each piece with a spoon
leaves from a small bunch
    of parsley, chopped
salt and pepper

I leave the skin on squash to act as a protective barrier, absorbing the full force of the flames' heat. It doesn't matter if it burns, as you can scrape the skin off, or pick a piece up and nibble the flesh away as if eating a slice of melon. Messy chops are all part of the barbecue experience.

Mix the garlic, cumin, chilli paste and oil in a large roasting tin. Lightly score the flesh sides of the butternut squash wedges with a sharp knife tip. Place them in the roasting tin, season well with salt and pepper, then turn them to coat in the marinade. Leave for 30 minutes while the barbecue reaches temperature.

Remove the squash from the tin and place the pieces directly on the grill over a medium heat, placing them flesh side-down first. Cook for 3–4 minutes on each flesh side, then turn them skin side-down and cook for a further 12 minutes, until the flesh is tender. If they look like they are cooking too fast, shift them to a cooler part of the grill.

When the pieces of squash are tender, scatter the parsley over the top and serve immediately.

SWEETCORN 'RIBS' WITH SHORT-CUT BARBECUE SAUCE

★

For the 'ribs'
4 sweetcorn cobs
olive oil
salt and pepper
lime wedges, to serve

For the sauce
6 tablespoons
   tomato ketchup
2 tablespoons brown sauce
1 tablespoon soy sauce
1 teaspoon smoked paprika
1 garlic clove,
   finely chopped

I first saw this dish made in a deep-fryer. The corn curls as it cooks, and that's what makes it resemble ribs. They'll work on a barbecue, too, they just need a nudge in a pan to start them off so they don't burn before they are cooked through. As for the barbecue sauce, there are plenty of recipes with a page-long list of ingredients, but this one is as fast as can be and relies on the components already having all the vinegar, sugar and spices that you need.

Light your barbecue!

While the flames are settling, boil a large saucepan of salted water. If the corn are still in their husks, strip them away. Boil the corn for 5 minutes, until partly cooked.

Meanwhile, make the sauce by mixing all the ingredients together in a bowl.

Cut each cob in quarters lengthways, including some of the core in each one. This can be tricky; a large sharp knife helps. Save the beer for after this part! Brush each 'rib' lightly with oil and season with salt and pepper.

Place the corn directly on the grid of your barbecue over a medium heat. Cook them for 6 minutes, until tender and nicely charred at the edges. They should curl slightly as they cook.

Brush them with half the sauce to glaze them, then cook for a final 2 minutes to let the sauce get sticky and dark.

Pile them on to a plate and serve with lime wedges for squeezing and the remaining sauce for dipping. Eat them immediately, gnawing the smoky kernels from the ribs.

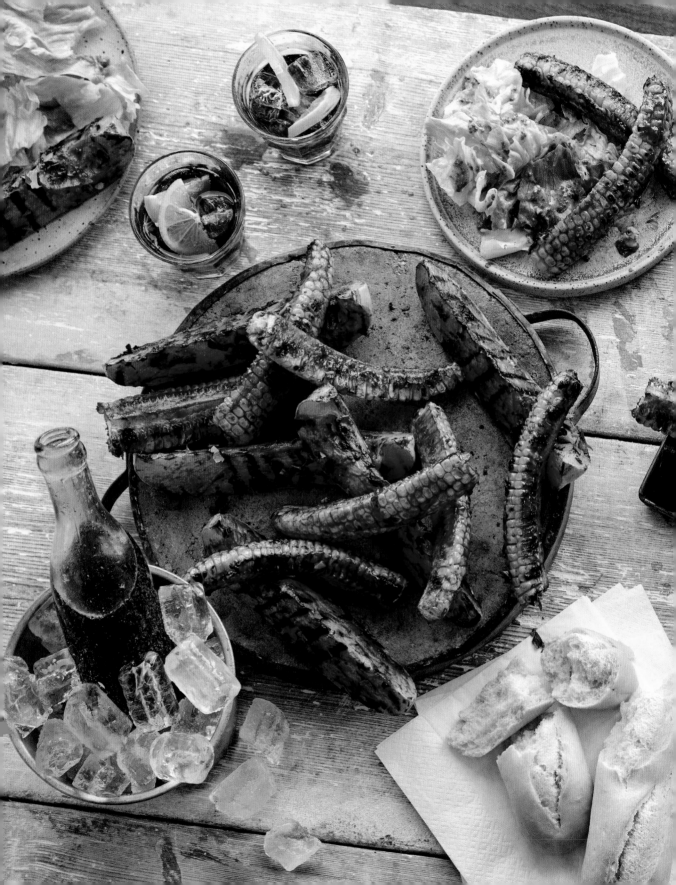

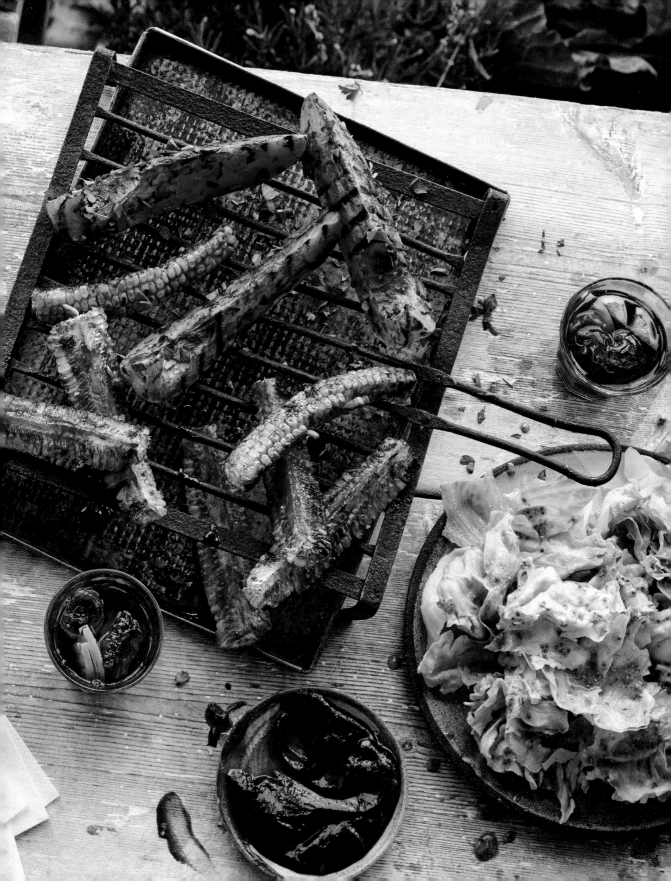

COURGETTE, RADISH, TOFU and SPRING ONION SKEWERS

★

2 courgettes
8 spring onions
400g packet firm tofu
16 radishes

For the marinade
**leaves from a small
bunch of oregano,
finely chopped**
**3 garlic cloves,
finely chopped**
juice of 1 lemon
olive oil
salt and pepper

*These need to be cooked over a medium-high direct heat.
The veg are all edible raw, so it doesn't matter if they still have
a bite to them. This marinade is a simple garlic and herb affair,
but you can use something more spicy if that's your thing.
You will need 8 bamboo or metal skewers.*

If you are using bamboo skewers, soak them in cold water for
20 minutes before using. This stops them bursting into flames.

Cut each courgette into 8 pieces. Trim each onion and cut them
into 3 equal pieces. Cut the tofu into 16 squares. Keep the radishes
whole, unless any are particularly large.

Thread an even mix of veg and tofu on to the skewers.

Mix the oregano, garlic and 1 tablespoon of lemon juice together
in a bowl. Add enough olive oil to give you a pesto-like paste,
then season with plenty of salt and pepper.

Place the skewers on to the barbecue over a high heat.
Cook for 8–10 minutes, until tender and coloured, turning
often. Start brushing and basting them with the marinade
halfway through cooking.

Finish with a squeeze of lemon juice. Eat immediately.

SOUTHERN SLAW
★

1 tablespoon mild mustard
2 tablespoons finely chopped
   gherkins, plus 1 tablespoon
   of their brine
2 tablespoons finely chopped
   pickled jalapenos, plus
   1 tablespoon of their brine
3 tablespoons vegan
   mayonnaise, or olive oil
¼ white cabbage
3 spring onions
1 large carrot
1 small fennel bulb
1 apple
2 tablespoons pumpkin seeds
2 teaspoons poppy seeds
small bunch of coriander
celery salt, to taste

A step beyond your everyday slaw. The gherkins and jalapenos add a hit of briny pickle, as does the mild-but-tangy mustard. There is sweetness from the apple and a bit of crunch from the seeds. I use French's mustard for this, but any hot dog mustard would work well. You could also use regular salt instead of the celery salt.

Mix the mustard, pickling liquids and mayonnaise or oil together in a mixing bowl.

Thinly shred the cabbage, thinly slice the spring onions and fennel, grate the carrot and dice the apple.

Add the gherkins, jalapenos and seeds to the veg. Finely chop the coriander (leaves only) and add to the bowl too. Mix well and season with celery salt, or regular salt, to taste.

CHOCOLATE BAKED BANANAS
★

4 bananas, cut lengthways
   but not all the way through
   (you just want to open up
   the skin on one side)
100g vegan dark
   chocolate buttons
4 shots of bourbon,
   whisky or rum

A campfire classic, boozy with Bourbon. A bed of glowing embers is perfect for tucking the bananas in to bake.

Push the chocolate buttons deep into the cuts, studding them the full length of each banana. Wrap each banana in foil, tipping a shot of booze into each just before sealing the foil edges together.

Place them into the embers of your fire and bake for 10 minutes, turning once. They'll look blackened and messy when you open them, but they'll smell and taste amazing. Open the parcel and use a spoon to scrape the chocolaty, boozy banana out of the skins.

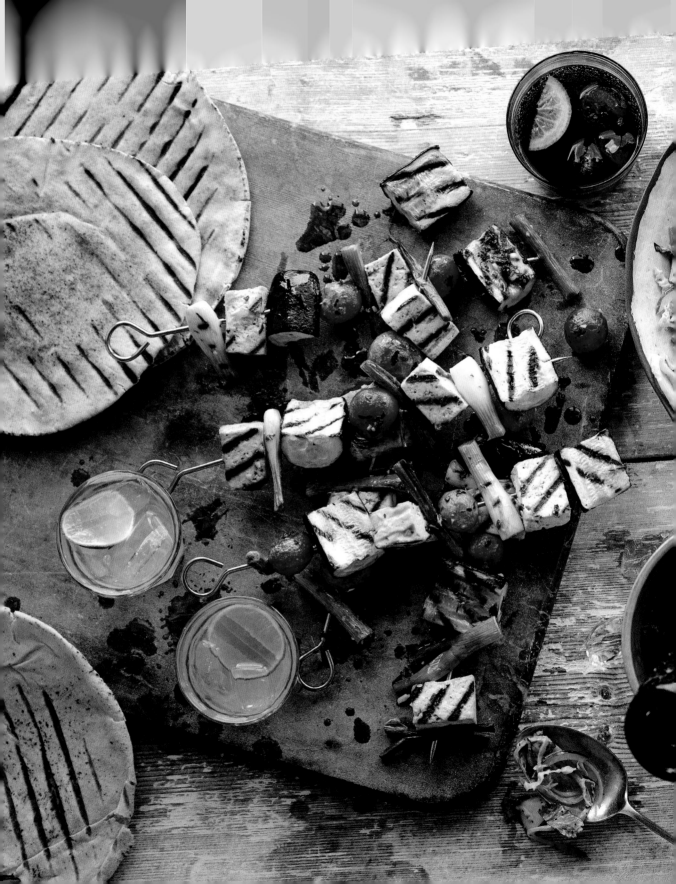

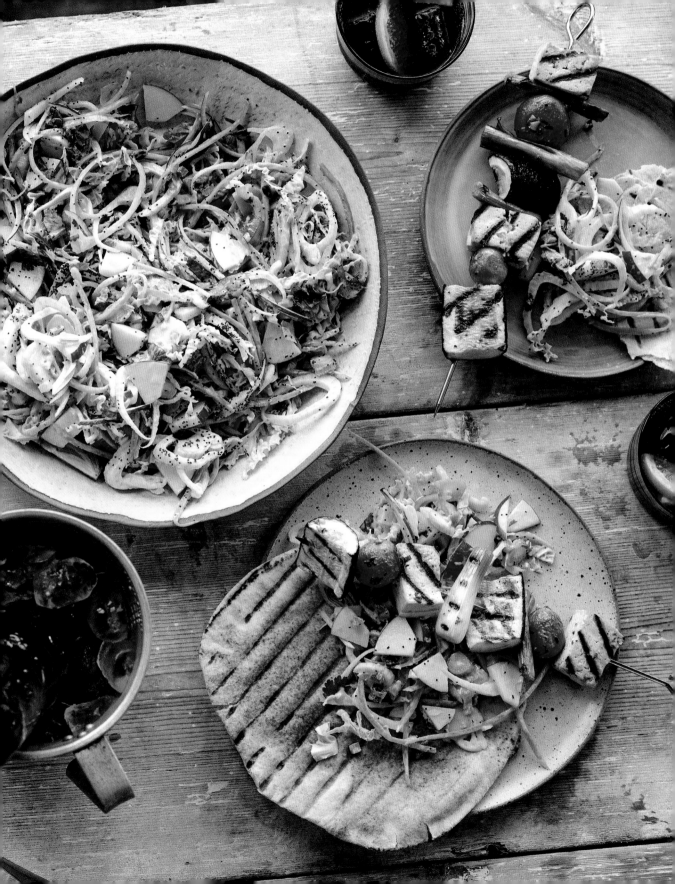

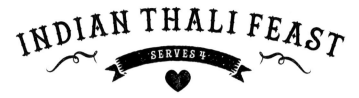

INDIAN THALI FEAST

SERVES 4

A thali is a collection of small dishes all brought together to make an epic meal. The way it works is that each person eating should get a little bit of each dish on their plate – kind of like tapas, but Indian, and all at once instead of on lots of little plates! It would be an effort to pull all of these together at one time, but plenty of the separate parts can be got ready in advance. Better still, get your mates each to be in charge of one dish and all come together over a few beers to sink the lot.

PREP: 15 MINUTES

CARROT and MANGO SALAD

★

2 large carrots
1 small or ½ large
    mango, skinned
    and finely chopped
½ tablespoon finely
    grated fresh root ginger
½ tablespoon black
    onion seeds
leaves from a small
    bunch of coriander,
    finely chopped
1 lime
salt

This is a fresh and simple side salad with a tropical hit to balance out the richer curries. I'd consider adding a bit of chilli and red onion, if there wasn't more than enough of both in the other dishes. If you have trouble finding a ripe mango, use a couple of tablespoons of mango chutney to dress the carrots instead.

Peel the carrots and use the vegetable peeler to pull them into thin ribbon-like pieces. Alternatively, coarsely grate them if you prefer.

Mix the carrot with the mango, ginger, black onion seeds and coriander. Season to taste with lime juice and salt.

ALOO MATAR

★

2 tablespoons coconut
or vegetable oil
1 red onion, finely chopped
1 teaspoon cumin seeds
½ tablespoon finely grated
fresh root ginger
2 garlic cloves,
finely chopped
1 teaspoon ground
coriander
½ teaspoon ground
turmeric
300g tomato passata
or chopped tomatoes
350g potatoes,
cut into 2cm cubes
2 green chillies
300ml water
100g frozen peas
1 teaspoon garam masala
chilli powder, to taste
(optional)
leaves from a small
bunch of coriander,
roughly chopped
salt and pepper

This sounds simple as it's just potatoes and peas, but the spices take it to another level. I like adding whole slit chillies to a curry – they release some of their heat into the dish, but nothing too aggressive. You can serve them to the person in the group who loves a hit of proper heat – usually me.

Heat the oil in a saucepan. Add the onion and fry over a medium heat for 5 minutes. Add the cumin seeds, ginger and garlic and cook for a further 2 minutes, stirring to make sure they don't stick.

Add the ground coriander, turmeric, passata or tomatoes and potatoes. Cut 4 lengthways slits into each of the green chillies and throw them in too, whole. Tip in the measured water and season well with salt and pepper.

Bring to the boil, then reduce the heat to a simmer and cook for 15 minutes, before adding the peas and cooking for a further 10 minutes, until the potatoes are tender and falling apart. Add a dash more water if it looks like drying out.

Stir in the garam masala. Taste and tweak the seasoning, adding some chilli powder for extra heat, if you like. Scatter with the coriander and serve.

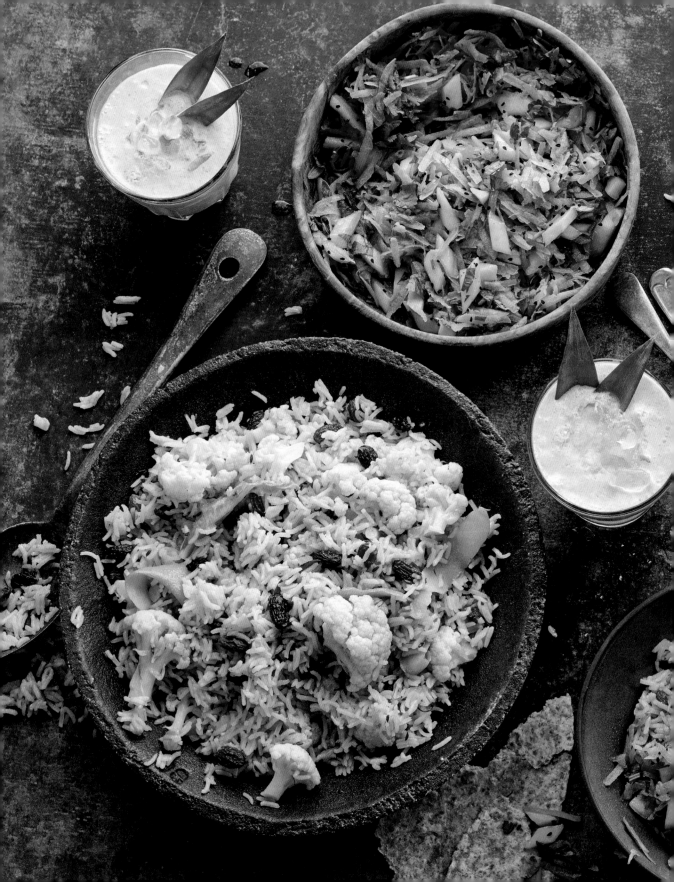

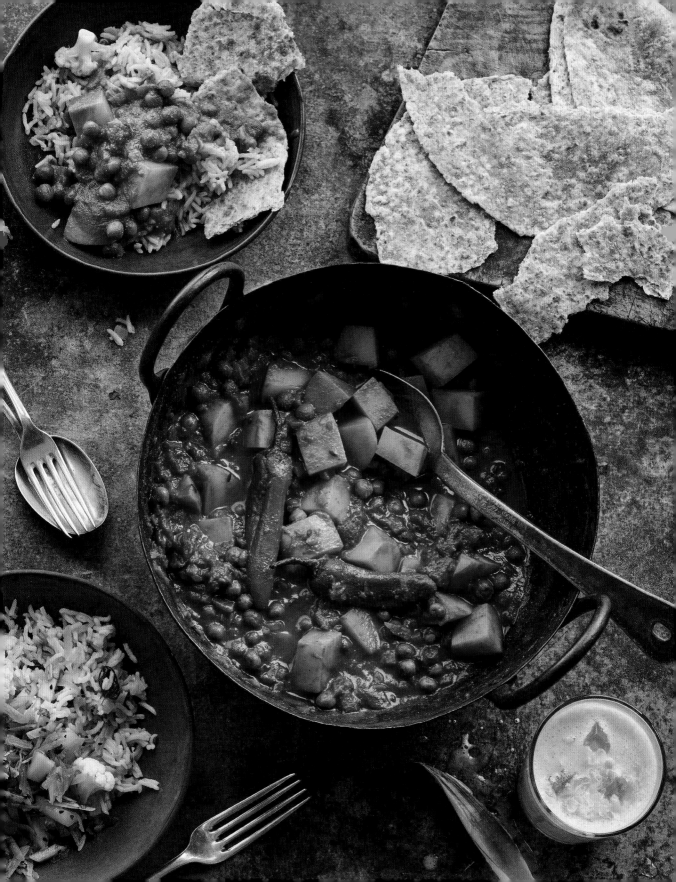

CAULIFLOWER PILAU RICE
★

3 tablespoons vegetable oil
1 onion, finely chopped
250g white basmati
    rice, rinsed
1 lemon
½ cauliflower, chopped
    into very small florets
40g raisins,
    roughly chopped
1 small cinnamon stick
pinch of saffron threads
1 teaspoon cumin seeds
2 bay leaves
100ml water
salt and pepper

I'm not using cauliflower instead of rice (which has been a bit trendy of late), but as well as rice. The cooking method here is a bit of a faff, but you'll be rewarded with light, fluffy, separate grains. Use a little ground turmeric in place of the saffron, if needs be.

Put a large saucepan of well-salted water on to boil.

Warm 1 tablespoon of the oil in a separate large saucepan. Add the onion and cook gently for 10 minutes, until starting to soften and colour.

Meanwhile, tip the drained rice into the boiling water. When it returns to the boil, reduce the heat and simmer for 5 minutes before draining well. Set aside.

Use a vegetable peeler to pull 4 long strips of zest from the lemon. Add them to the onion along with the cauliflower florets, raisins, cinnamon, saffron, cumin, bay and 2 more tablespoons of oil. Season with salt and pepper and fry gently for 2 minutes.

Tip the measured water into the pan and gently fold in the rice. Level it out with a wooden spoon, trying not to compress it too much. Use the handle of the spoon to poke 12 holes in the rice – this allows the steam to move through it.

Place a clean tea towel on top of the saucepan and place the lid on top. Fold the edges of the cloth up and over the lid so they can't catch on the hob – a kitchen fire would put a downer on your evening. Reduce the heat to as low as you possibly can and cook for 20 minutes. The rice should be tender, light and fluffy and just beginning to catch on the pan.

Taste and tweak the seasoning with salt, pepper and a squeeze or so of lemon juice, if needed.

CHICKPEAS and COCONUT
★

400g can chickpeas,
    liquid included
½ x 400g can coconut milk
salt
2 tablespoons toasted
    coconut flakes (optional)

For the curry paste
2 dried chillies
seeds from 4
    cardamom pods
1 teaspoon cumin seeds
1 teaspoon coriander seeds
1 tablespoon finely grated
    fresh root ginger
2 garlic cloves,
    finely chopped
¼ teaspoon ground
    cinnamon
1 teaspoon ground turmeric
40g cashew nuts
juice of ½ lemon
2 tablespoons coconut
    or vegetable oil

If this curry paste has a name I don't know it, but it works on so many things and you can use it as a base for any mixture of pulses or veg. This chickpea version couldn't be simpler. I almost called it chickpea mash, as you want them to turn soft and begin to fall apart as the sauce thickens around them.

In a small food processor or blender, blitz all the curry paste ingredients together. Alternatively bash them into a paste in a mortar and pestle.

Put a saucepan over a medium heat and fry the paste for a few minutes, until it's smelling fragrant. Keep stirring and make sure it doesn't catch.

Tip in the chickpeas and their liquid, followed by the coconut milk. Season with salt and simmer gently for 25 minutes, until the chickpeas are very soft and the sauce is thick. Add a dash of water if it looks like drying out at any point.

Taste and tweak with more salt, if needed. Sprinkle with the coconut flakes, if you fancy.

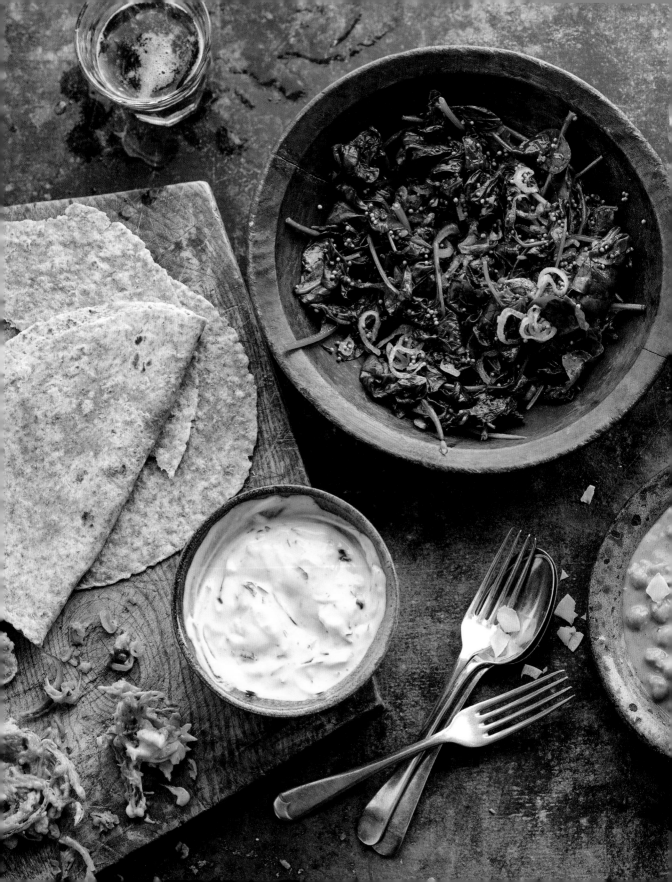

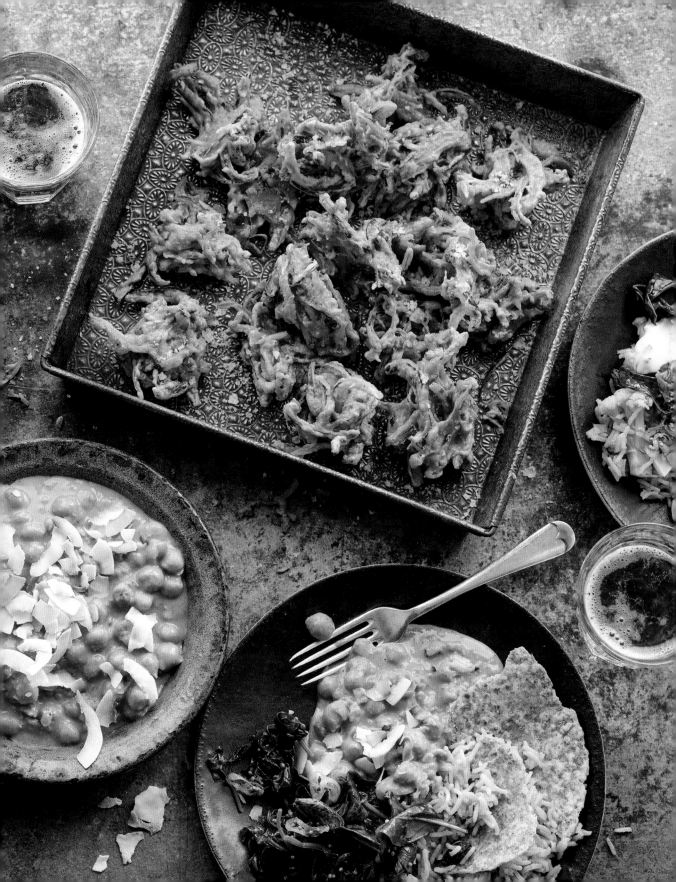

TARKA SPINACH
★

400g spinach
3 tablespoons coconut oil
2 shallots, thinly sliced
1 tablespoon curry leaves
1 teaspoon mustard seeds
1 teaspoon cumin seeds
salt and pepper

Tarka is a fried spice mix that is usually used to finish a dhal. I'm using it here to add some pop to a simple side of spinach.

Wash your spinach well and strip out and discard any particularly coarse stalks.

Heat the oil in a saucepan and add the shallots. Fry over a medium-high heat for 2 minutes, until they are starting to colour. Throw in the curry leaves, mustard seeds and cumin seeds. Cook for a couple more minutes, until the mustard seeds start to pop.

Stir in the spinach until just wilted, it will only take a couple of minutes. Season with salt and pepper to finish.

PREP: 10 MINUTES

RAITA

½ cucumber
200g unsweetened
  vegan natural yogurt
leaves from a small
  bunch of mint,
  thinly sliced
salt

There are plenty of coconut-based vegan yogurts on the market that would be ideal for this dish.

Deseed the cucumber by halving it lengthways, then removing the seeds with the tip of a teaspoon. Discard them. Coarsely grate the cucumber and squeeze out some of its excess water with your hands (you could wrap it in a clean tea towel for this part).

Mix the cucumber into the yogurt along with the mint. Taste and season with salt, erring on the generous side, to taste.

ONION and LIME PICKLE BHAJIS

★

100g gram (chickpea) flour
100ml water
sunflower or vegetable oil,
    for deep-frying
2 tablespoons lime pickle
½ teaspoon ground
    turmeric
leaves from a small
    bunch of coriander,
    finely chopped
2 red onions, thinly sliced
salt

A classic bhaji pepped up with the king of curry house condiments. No need for a complex list of herbs and spices, the pickle brings it all to the party, along with its mouth-puckering sourness.

Whisk the chickpea flour and measured water in a mixing bowl with a generous pinch of salt until there are no lumps.

Get a heavy, deep-sided saucepan and add the oil until it is 6–8cm deep, you don't want it to be more than one-third full for safety reasons. Slowly bring the oil up to 180°C, over a medium heat. Either use a thermometer to check the temperature, or use the handle of a wooden spoon: dip it in and you want to see steady bubbling around it. If there's loads of lively bubbles, the oil is too hot; too few and it's not hot enough. (This is important as cool oil will give you greasy bhajis, but very hot oil will burn them before they are cooked through.)

While the oil heats up, put the lime pickle on a chopping board and chop it into a coarse paste. Add it to the gram flour batter with the turmeric, coriander and onions. Mix together and taste, to check the seasoning, tweaking with a little more salt if necessary.

When the oil is ready, shape clumsy balls of the mixture in a tablespoon and drop them carefully into the pan. Don't put more than 4 in at a time, or the oil temperature will drop too much. Fry for 3–4 minutes, until golden, crisp and buoyant.

Remove carefully with a slotted spoon and drain on kitchen paper to soak up any oil, while you fry the rest in batches in the same way. Scoff hot!

ACKNOWLEDGEMENTS

This book would not have been possible without the help and input of the following people. Rob (Bob) Andrew for all the recipes he's put into this book along with his experience, help and advice. Rachel Lovell for all of her hard work with Dirty Vegan and helping get this book together. Dale Templar and Owen Gay from One Tribe TV productions. Designers Alex and Emma Smith and the amazing photography teams of Chris Terry and Jamie Orlando Smith, as well as food stylist Phil Mundy and props stylist Olivia Wardle. Fun times taking the pics for this book, especially the cabbages and our day in Cardiff (burn him). Everyone at One Tribe Talent and One Tribe TV productions. All the team at Octopus books. Thanks to Adam El Tagoury from Anna Loka café in Cardiff. Big thanks to Laura from Tidy Kitchen who has been a star and has also contributed a guest recipe so I hope you enjoy it. Thanks also to Kelsey for her chiffon cake. Also a guest recipe from my mate Pancho. He always enjoyed cooking so I asked him if he'd like to add his tacos to the book. He was up for it and they taste delish, so cheers, Panch.

Just a big thanks to all really for your continued help and support.

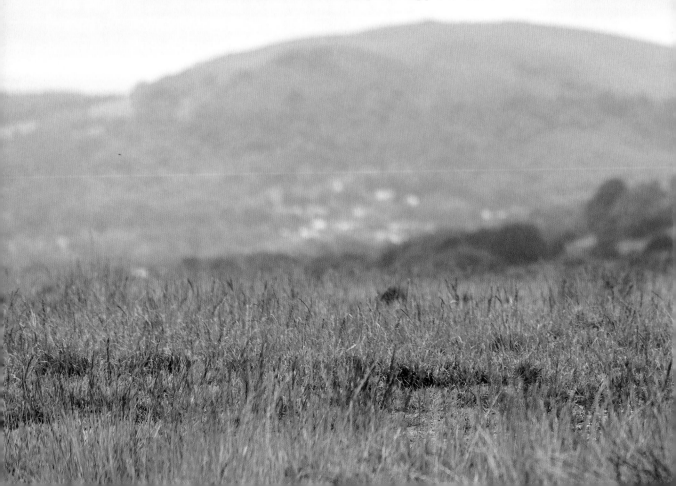

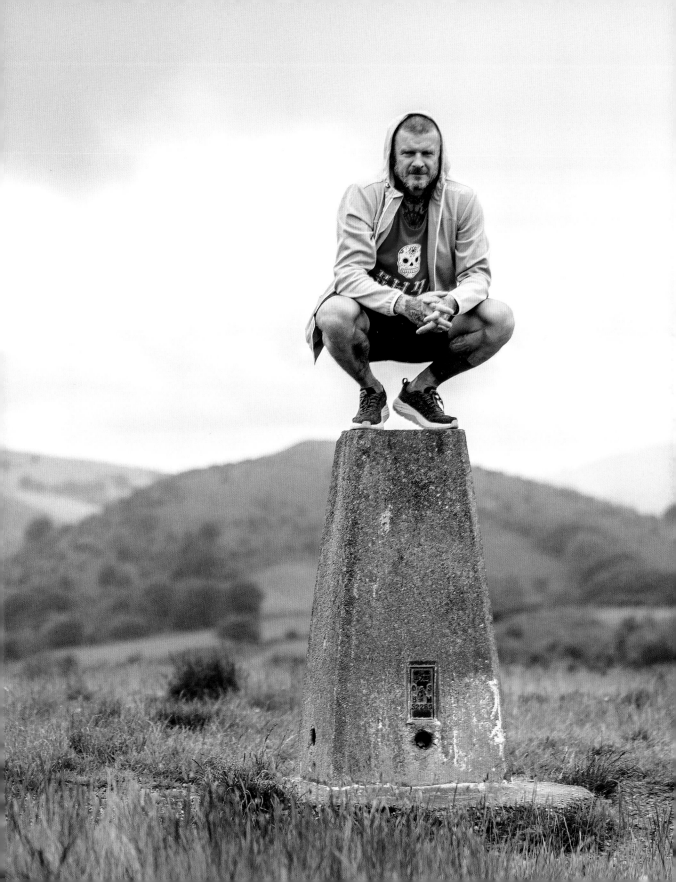

INDEX

★

A

ackee, jerk sweet potato stew 54–5
aloo matar 193
apples
    apple and blackberry
        cobbler 150
    apple, maple and cinnamon
        doughnuts 138
asparagus
    asparagus 'cheese' straws 171
    freekeh stinger fritters 65–6
    minty courgettes with popped
        beans and tahini 56
    whipped white bean and
        asparagus toasts 104
aubergines
    baby aubergine, chickpea
        and olive tagine 36
    caponata with borlotti
        beans 44
avocados
    chocolate avo mousse 131
    power hit salad bowl 118
    Tex Mex quinoa salad with
        avocado dressing 102

B

báhn mì with tempeh
    and green pâté 100
bananas
    chocolate baked bananas 189
    chocolate and olive oil 148
    a pair of banana breads 147
bao buns, sticky tofu 109–10
barbecue feast 184–9
barley, penny bun, black
        kale and barley
        stew 67
beans
    báhn mì with tempeh
        and green pâté 100

caponata with borlotti beans 44
frijoles 166
green tabbouleh 174
jerk sweet potato stew 54–5
la-la-lasagne 94
leek, spinach and white
    bean pies 34
minty courgettes with popped
    beans and tahini 56
Peking crispy jackfruit
    pancakes 28
power hit salad bowl 118
smokey-sheezy-garlicky
    pasta 76
Tex Mex quinoa salad with
    avocado dressing 102
whipped white bean and
    asparagus toasts 104
beetroot
    beetroot and red wine
        risotto 18
    beetroot, spinach and
        mushroom Wellington 179
    brined and barbecued
        rainbow root veg 80
    roast beetroot and smoked
        tofu salad 116
    Scandi beetroot, potato
        and fennel salad 46
blackberries, apple and
    blackberry cobbler 150
boneless broth three
        ways 121
chocolate baked bananas 189
broccoli
    rocking cauli and
        banging broccoli 111
    satay broccoli with
        crispy onions 62
    smokey-sheezy-garlicky
        pasta 76

Brussel sprouts, sprouts,
    cabbage and chestnuts
    with crispy garlic 181
bulgur wheat, green
    tabbouleh 174

C

cabbage
    Southern slaw 189
    sprouts, cabbage and chestnuts
        with crispy garlic 181
caponata with borlotti beans 44
carrots
    carrot and herb pakoras
        with mango and herb
        chutney 89–90
    carrot and mango salad 192
    fast falafel with carrot salad
        and harissa tahini 22
    harira 112
    parsnips and carrots with
        clementines and spices 178
    Southern slaw 189
    vegan Irish stew 72
    winter root Caesar salad
        with crispy capers 52
cauliflower
    cauliflower fattoush 106
    cauliflower pilau rice 196
    Pancho's tacos 38
    rocking cauli and banging
        broccoli 111
chestnuts, sprouts, cabbage
    and chestnuts with crispy
    garlic 181
chickpeas
    baby aubergine, chickpea
        and olive tagine 36
    chickpeas and coconut 197
    fast falafel with carrot salad
        and harissa tahini 22

harira 112
power hit salad bowl 118
chilli non carne tempeh
    tostadas 163
chocolate
    chocolate baked bananas 189
    chocolate avo mousse 131
    chocolate cinder toffee 134
    chocolate dippers 138
    chocolate and olive oil 148
    chocolate orange chiffon
        cake 129–30
    puffed pears with chocolate
        and olive oil sauce 154–5
Christmas feast 178–81
Christmas pud, Pritch's 141–2
courgettes
    caponata with borlotti
        beans 44
    fast and furious soy
        and sriracha stir-fry
        with rice 32
    green tabbouleh 174
    courgette, radish, tofu
        and spring onion
        skewers 188
    minty courgettes with
        popped beans and
        tahini 56
    one-pot courgette, pea
        and spinach pasta 20
    stuffed courgette flowers
        with tomatoes and
        farro 58–9
    wok 'n' roll stir-fry 86
cucumber, kiwi, cucumber
    and lime ice lollies 146

D
dial-it-up brown lentil dhal 95
doughnuts 136–9

F
farro, stuffed courgette
    flowers with tomatoes
    and farro 58–9
fennel

beetroot and red wine risotto 18
Scandi beetroot, potato
    and fennel salad 46
Southern slaw 189
freekeh stinger fritters 65–6
frijoles 166
fruit ice lollies 145–7

G
gazpacho 170
gravy 122
green rice 167
green tabbouleh 174

H
harira 112

I
ice lollies 145–7
Indian Thali feast 192–201
Irish stew, vegan 72

J
jackfruit, Peking crispy
    jackfruit pancakes 28
jam doughnuts 138
jerk sweet potato stew 54–5

K
kale
    baked squash speltotto 60
    penny bun, black kale
        and barley stew 67
    winter root Caesar salad
        with crispy capers 52
katsu curry, tofu 16
kiwifruit
    kiwi, cucumber and lime
        ice lollies 146
    planty panna cotta with
        kiwifruit sauce 132

L
la-la-lasagne 94
leeks
    leek, spinach and white
        bean pies 34

rainbow chard, leek
    and lentil gratin 50
lentils
    beetroot, spinach and
        mushroom Wellington 179
    dial-it-up brown lentil dhal 95
    harira 112
    lentil Sloppy Joes 85
    porcini shepherd's pie 78
    rainbow chard, leek
        and lentil gratin 50
lettuce
    cauliflower fattoush 106
    freekeh stinger fritters 65–6
    salad soup with wild
        garlic pesto 114
    Thai tempeh larb salad
        with rice cake
        croutons 48
limes, kiwi, cucumber and
    lime ice lollies 146

M
mangoes
    carrot and herb pakoras
        with mango and herb
        chutney 89–90
    carrot and mango
        salad 192
    Pancho's tacos 38
    pineapple, mango and
        coconut ice lollies 145
Mexican feast 162–7
mushrooms
    beetroot, spinach and
        mushroom Wellington 179
    better-than sausage
        rolls 91–2
    creamy mushroom
        pritchanoff 74–5
    la-la-lasagne 94
    mushroom ragu with
        polenta 26
    penny bun, black kale
        and barley stew 67
    porcini shepherd's pie 78
    vegan Irish stew 72

N

nettles, freekeh stinger
fritters 65–6

O

olives
baby aubergine, chickpea
and olive tagine 36
caponata with borlotti
beans 44
cashew nuts 83
popeye pie 83–4
stuffed courgette flowers
with tomatoes and
farro 58–9
oranges
chocolate orange chiffon
cake 129–30
Pritch's Christmas pud 141–2
raspberry friands 143
Scandi beetroot, potato
and fennel salad 46

P

Pancho's tacos 38
parsnips
parsnips and carrots with
clementines and spices 178
vegan Irish stew 72
winter root Caesar salad
with crispy capers 52
pasta
one-pot courgette, pea
and spinach pasta 20
smokey-sheezy-garlicky
pasta 76
peaches, Turkish delight
barbecue peaches 152
pearl barley, better-than
sausage rolls 91–2
pears, puffed pears with
chocolate and olive oil
sauce 154–5
peas
aloo matar 193
báhn mì with tempeh
and green pâté 100

fast and furious soy and
sriracha stir-fry with rice 32
freekeh stinger fritters 65–6
one-pot courgette, pea
and spinach pasta 20
salad soup with wild
garlic pesto 114
Peking crispy jackfruit
pancakes 28
penny bun, black kale
and barley stew 67
peppers
gazpacho 170
green rice 167
jerk sweet potato stew 54–5
piri-piri tempeh tray bake
with sweet potato wedges 30
Tex Mex quinoa salad with
avocado dressing 102
wok 'n' roll stir-fry 86
picnic feast 170–5
pineapple, mango and
coconut ice lollies 145
piri-piri tempeh tray bake
with sweet potato wedges 30
planty panna cotta with
kiwifruit sauce 132
polenta
mushroom ragu
with polenta 26
polenta and rosemary
roasties 180
popeye pie 83–4
porcini shepherd's pie 78
potatoes
aloo matar 193
polenta and rosemary
roasties 180
porcini shepherd's pie 78
potato and onion tortilla 175
power hit salad bowl 118
salad soup with wild
garlic pesto 114
Scandi beetroot, potato
and fennel salad 46
vegan Irish stew 72
power hit salad bowl 118

Pritchard's dressing 118
Pritch's Christmas pud 141–2

Q

quinoa, Tex Mex quinoa salad
with avocado dressing 102

R

rainbow chard, leek
and lentil gratin 50
raita 200
raspberry friands 143
rhubarb and custard
doughnuts 138
rice
beetroot and red wine
risotto 18
cauliflower pilau rice 196
creamy mushroom
pritchanoff 74–5
fast and furious soy and
sriracha stir-fry with rice 32
green rice 167
harira 112
tofu katsu curry 16
rice cakes, Thia tempeh larb
salad with rice cake
croutons 48
rice noodles, roasting tin laksa 24
rocking cauli and banging
broccoli 111

S

salad soup with wild garlic
pesto 114
salsa, chopped 162
satay broccoli with crispy
onions 62
Scandi beetroot, potato
and fennel salad 46
smokey, pokey sweetcorn
and spinach chowder 120
Southern slaw 189
spelt, baked squash speltotto 60
spinach
beetroot, spinach and
mushroom Wellington 179

green rice 167
jerk sweet potato stew 54–5
leek, spinach and white
    bean pies 34
one-pot courgette, pea
    and spinach pasta 20
popeye pie 83–4
power hit salad bowl 118
smokey, pokey sweetcorn
    and spinach chowder 120
tarka spinach 200
spring onions
    freekeh stinger fritters 65–6
    courgette, radish, tofu
        and spring onion
        skewers 188
    jerk sweet potato
        stew 54–5
    salad soup with wild
        garlic pesto 114
    Southern slaw 189
    Thai tempeh larb salad
        with rice cake croutons 48
    wok 'n' roll stir-fry 86
squash
    baked squash speltotto 60
    roasting tin laksa 24
    spicy smokey squash 184
strawberries, strawberry,
    watermelon and basil
    ice lollies 146
swede, vegan Irish stew 72
sweet potatoes
    jerk sweet potato stew 54–5
    lentil Sloppy Joes 85
    piri-piri tempeh tray bake
        with sweet potato
        wedges 30
sweetcorn
    Pancho's tacos 38
    smokey, pokey sweetcorn
        and spinach chowder 120
    sweetcorn 'ribs' with short-cut
        barbecue sauce 185
    Tex Mex quinoa salad with
        avocado dressing 102
    wok 'n' roll stir-fry 86

T
tempeh
    báhn mì with tempeh
        and green pâté 100
    chilli non carne tempeh
        tostadas 163
    piri-piri tempeh tray
        bake with sweet
        potato wedges 30
    Thai tempeh larb
        salad with rice cake
        croutons 48
Tenderstem broccoli
    leek, spinach and white
        bean pies 34
    Peking crispy jackfruit
        pancakes 28
Tex Mex quinoa salad with
    avocado dressing 102
Thai tempeh larb
    salad with rice cake
    croutons 48
tofu
    courgette, radish, tofu
        and spring onion
        skewers 188
    popeye pie 83, 83–4
    roast beetroot and smoked
        tofu salad 116
    smokey-sheezy-garlicky
        pasta 76
    sticky tofu bao buns 109–10
    tofu katsu curry 16
tomatoes
    cauliflower fattoush 106
    chopped salsa 162
    gazpacho 170
    green tabbouleh 174
    jerk sweet potato stew 54–5
    piri-piri tempeh tray
        bake with sweet
        potato wedges 30
    porcini shepherd's pie 78
    power hit salad bowl 118
    stuffed courgette flowers
        with tomatoes and
        farro 58–9

Tex Mex quinoa salad
    with avocado dressing 102
tortillas
    chilli non carne tempeh
        tostadas 163
    Pancho's tacos 38
    Turkish delight barbecue
        peaches 152

V
vegan cheese
    asparagus 'cheese' straws 171
    la-la-lasagne 94
vegan Irish stew 72
vegetable stock 121

W
watermelon, strawberry,
    watermelon and basil
    ice lollies 146
whipped white bean and
    asparagus toasts 104
wild garlic, salad soup
    with wild garlic pesto 114
winter root Caesar salad
    with crispy capers 52
wok 'n' roll stir-fry 86

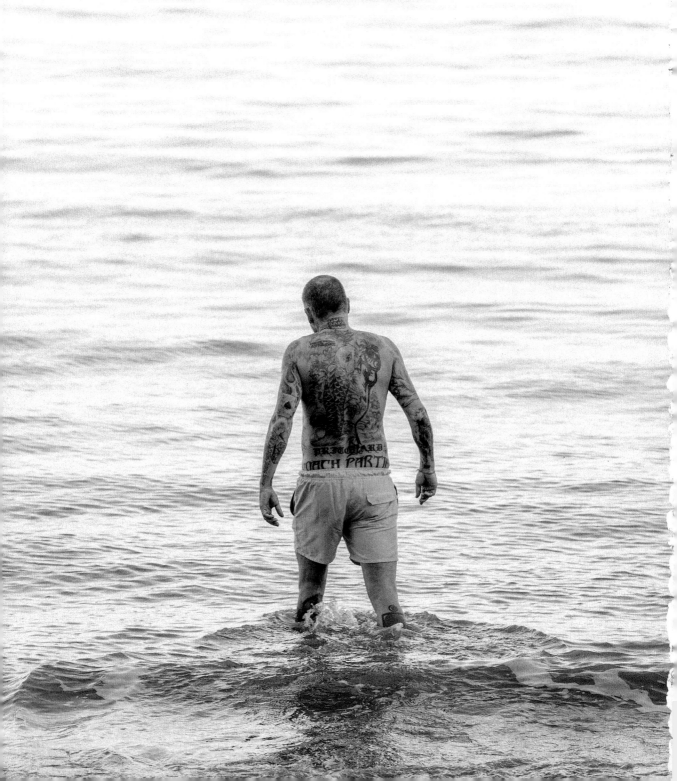